DON'T DIET.
BE HAPPY.

Don't Diet Be Happy
Copyright © 2022 by Katherine McIntosh
ISBN: 978-1-63493-600-2

All rights reserved. No part of this publication may be reproduced, stored in a retrieval system, or transmitted, in any form or by any means electronic, mechanical, photocopying, recording, or otherwise without prior written permission from the publisher.

The author and publisher of the book do not make any claim or guarantee for any physical, mental, emotional, spiritual, or financial result. All products, services and information provided by the author are for general education and entertainment purposes only.
The information provided herein is in no way a substitute for medical advice. In the event you use any of the information contained in this book for yourself, the author and publisher assume no responsibility for your actions.

Published by Access Consciousness® Publishing
Cover and interior design by: Zoe Norvell

Don't Diet.
Be Happy.

Creating the
Body, Business, & Life
You Love

Katherine McIntosh

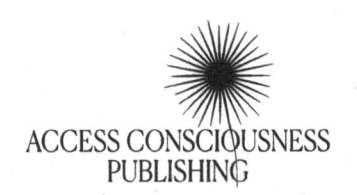

ACCESS CONSCIOUSNESS
PUBLISHING

Dedication

To my son Duke:

Since before you were born, you have always been an inspiration, inviting everyone in the world to see their beauty and believe in themselves. You are the catalyst behind this movement. You came at a perfect time in my life, and I am so grateful to walk this earth with you. I wouldn't be where I am without you. Thank you for the gift you continue to be to me and to the world.

I also dedicate this book to all the people who have spent their lives trying to change their bodies, to all the ones who thought you weren't enough just the way you are…

For those who are constantly on a diet, or thinking about a diet, or talking about how you just need to lose 5 pounds. For those who have been talking about it forever. This is for you.

I dedicate this book to those who are constantly trying to follow the rules when it comes to their bodies—from diets to gym memberships to green drinks to pills—but it never actually works...and worse, it never actually makes you feel good. To those who wake up and judge themselves, who think that something is wrong with you because you just can't seem to have the body you really want. This is for you.

This is your wake up call.

And finally, I dedicate this book to the beauty in all of us. It is more than skin deep and it's time to let it shine, both inside and out. Your beauty, your joy, and your happiness changes you, your body, and your life. Focus on your creations and everything in your life can grow.

Acknowledgment

This book and where my life is today would not have been possible without the contribution of so many individuals along the way. These include my parents, siblings, school teachers, college professors, energy workers, healers, coaches, children, mentors, friends, relationships, and co-workers. I am particularly grateful to the people who have helped this book in every evolution of its process (more on these individuals below).

Additionally, there are two individuals who deserve particular accolades of gratitude and adoration: Gary Douglas and Dr. Dain Heer. These two brilliant, courageous, generous men opened up my world to a way of being I always dreamed of but never knew was possible.

I learned that life doesn't have to be hard. Gary and Dain: Thank you for never giving up on what you saw was possible. Thank you for bringing your gifts to the world. In a time of great change, they are needed now more than ever. Thank you for encouraging me, inspiring me, and inviting me to know what I know. I would not be here without your perseverance and desire to change the world.

To all my amazing teachers, friends, healers, coaches, and mentors, thank you for educating me, inspiring me, and inviting me to the knowledge that changed my life every step of the way.

To my mom, thank you for always being there in the good times and the bad times. You picked me up from the ashes when I was falling apart and not many others were there. You never expected anything in return. Your unconditional love and support has meant the world to me. Thank you for always teaching me what it means to be kind, to treat others with respect, and to never give up on your dreams no matter what.

Finally, to all the amazing beings who contributed to the birth, institution, and growth of this book, thank you for seeing the vision, inspiring the movement, and being a catalyst for a greater reality. My goal is to live in a world where people stop judging their bodies. You always believed in this movement. Your personal contributions have been a gift. You are the change makers. Thank you for inspiring me.

Special acknowledgment to: Michelle Lylle, Lindsay Prince, Sandy Olson, Maureen Malloy, Rebecca Hulse, Emily Evans Russell, Will Williams, Janelle Forbes, Za Harustaran, Ashley McCaughey, Justin Cadrain, Nikki Martin, Christine Ciona, Stacey Paciencia, Alyssa Falk, Alexandra Roeth, Patty Alfonso, Rachel O'Brien, Megan Hill, Simone Milasis, Brendan Watt, Heather Nichols, Alun Jones, Peggy Sue Honeymoon Scott, Ilham Ouzani, Seve LeTour, Jenny Frithiof, Adriana Maya, Chris Woods, Jenilynne Coley, Christine McCarthy, Dr. Glenna Rice, Dr. Don Hemerson, Andrea Leger, Heather Coon, Deborah Newby, Heather Lawson, Stelian Busuioc Trina Rice, Katie Landers at The West End Med Spa, Rene Rose, Rose Jeans, Cecilia Villareal, and all the translators all over the world who continue to share and carry on this message, and so many others who haven't been named. Hopefully, you know who you are.

Thank you for believing in me.

What else is possible now?

Table of Contents

Author's Note	1
Introduction	15
Chapter 1: My Closet Nightmare	27
Chapter 2: Your Reflection Isn't Real	41
Chapter 3: The Birth of No Judgment Diet™	49
Chapter 4: The Beginning of Something Different	59
Chapter 5: Go On a Date... with Your Body!	71
Chapter 6: Wake Up Every Day As If You Just Met Your Body!	97
Chapter 7: Be Curious And Ask Questions! The Power Of A Question	111
Chapter 8: Have Gratitude For What Your Body Can Do!	125
Chapter 9: Play!	137
Chapter 10: Be Excited!	149
Chapter 11: Let Go Of Conclusions!	163
Chapter 12: Follow The Lightness	171
Chapter 13: Turn Yourself On!	183
Chapter 14: Your Body's Way	189
Appendix	195
About The Author	197

Author's Note

There I was on the couch in my living room with a raging male teenager hovering over me like an ape hovers over its prey, pressing a shiny silver blade up against my carotid. At first, I thought it was a joke, but when I looked at the frothing anger inside his eyes, I realized I was facing a life or death scenario. I panicked and started to shake, tremble, and scream. Luckily, the piercing volume of my screams shocked my brother to his core and for a brief moment, it was enough for me to free myself from his raging grasp. I ran as fast as I could, grabbed the phone, and locked myself in our downstairs bathroom. At first, I thought I was safe, but then the pounding sound of a butcher's knife trying to break through the solid wood door had me, with trembling hands, fumbling to keep my fingers steady enough to press the buttons - 9 - 1 - 1. As I waited for the sound of sirens, I could hear my heart beating through my chest, and feel the panting from the realization that in a flash, I came close to possibly losing my life.

At 17 years old, in a fit of rage, my 14-year-old brother put a butcher's knife to my throat. That incident radically and forever changed the dynamics of life as I knew it. Growing up in a rather dysfunctional family, I learned to pretend everything was fine. But the truth was, and I didn't discover this til later in life, (especially while studying to get my Master's in Somatic Psychology) my life, and my upbringing was anything but fine. My sweet, amazing, hard-working mother tried desperately to uphold this unrealistic image of a Happy Irish Catholic Family (an oxymoron), but when a slew of cop cars showed up in front of our driveway & took my brother away in our upper-middle-class neighborhood, the barely held together image started to crumble along with the rest of us.

My fragile and tumultuous teenage years were a mix of fending for myself and being forced to take on responsibilities older and more mature than my age. I was completely estranged from the idea of family; and yet, I felt tied by obligation, as the oldest, to set the example. Looking back at those times in my life, it was a bit much for me. I had to grow up quicker than I was ready for. I found relief on the soccer field, volleyball court, and ski hill, and I spent hours practicing my craft and drowning out the pain of what felt like a big gaping hole of shame in my universe.

I looked around at my friend's families and they genuinely seemed happy. There were no slamming doors, late-night fights, family secrets, unrealistic expectations, and absentee parents. I was jealous because I so badly wanted a normal life. I spent 20 years of my life hating my body and spending most of my life desperately searching for something that would fill this giant gaping hole inside me.

My life experiences, although not easy, have led me to be the strong, willful, determined being I am today. And that, I don't regret. But most people, when I tell the stories of my life, they cannot believe what I put myself through.

I don't tell my stories to make you feel sorry for me, or to paint myself as a victim. I tell my stories in hopes that it empowers you to find the strength within to live your BEST life, no matter what your story is. I believe that we truly create everything in our lives, whether it is conscious or unconscious, our spirit guides us to the lessons we need to learn until we learn them.

Going back to that fateful spring day after arriving home from a hard-earned victorious soccer match, having cop cars arrive on the scene shortly after my close encounter with death, was not in the plans. As my mom arrived home, the unexpected scene in front of her house shocked and frightened her. She didn't mean to at the time, but in the sheer terror that rippled through her body in that moment when the rest of her life was falling apart, she lost it and blamed me for the entire incident.

I couldn't handle it. I had almost lost my life and I was getting blamed for it! No way. I immediately packed my bags and moved out. Moving out was extremely taboo and went against everything we were taught as kids, which was appearances were more important than the truth. I didn't realize it at the time, but this would cause me to make life choices that were never really in my best interest.

I went to live with my best friend and her Latin family and had one of the best summers I had experienced because, for the first time in my entire life, I finally felt free from the heaviness of what was happening in the house I grew up in. I also got to experience what it was like to live with and be a part of a family that was kind, generous, fun-loving, and real. There was no pretending and no hiding. It was a radical contrast to my own upbringing and made me realize that the trauma I had endured most of my life was NOT normal.

For the first time in my life, I felt safe. As fall approached, I knew I would have to go back home, be in my school district, and face the harsh reality of my dysfunctional life. Against my need to feel safe and be a part of a family I didn't want to leave, I forced myself to move back in with my own family so I could continue to play soccer with my state-winning championship soccer team. Moving back into an environment where I didn't feel safe was just the beginning of developing an extremely tumultuous relationship with my body.

I didn't really think anything of it at the time. I just pressed on, but the truth is, that one decision to move back home, literally kept me in fight or flight my entire senior year. I had no idea how unsafe I felt and how much feeling unsafe would not only destroy my fit, athletic body, but it would also destroy my ability to make long-term healthy life choices. I would come home from soccer practice, grab food, lock myself in my bedroom, eat by myself, and do everything I could to avoid family interactions.

If I ate dinner with the family, I would eat as fast as possible and then I wouldn't stop until I was numb. I did anything to try to drown out the pain that left me hollow to my core. With a shattered nervous system, my body could no longer handle the stresses, process food properly, or maintain a strong, healthy metabolism.

My body became the enemy and I drowned myself in self-pity every time I looked in the mirror. I couldn't see the sparkly green-eyed fit athlete. Instead, I could only see the depressed shell of a being and when I looked in the mirror the reflection staring back at me was FAT.

I honestly didn't realize how much my nervous system was in constant fight or flight. So no matter how much or how little I ate, I eventually gained over 20 pounds my senior year in high school. The trauma didn't allow my body to digest food properly and it was in constant survival mode.

That experience was the beginning of a lifelong struggle of yo-yo-ing from 126 pounds to 145 pounds to 115 pounds to 150 pounds to 165 pounds to 130 pounds to 96 pounds and more. I literally went up and down, and up and down, and up and down for over 20 years. It was hell. I hated myself for it.

No matter what my weight was, I never felt good about myself and I never truly loved the skin I was in. I spent most of my adult life desperate to love my body. So even if I seemed happy on the outside, the truth is, I was always looking out for the next thing that would promise to help me lose weight. I thought If I could change the outside that the inside would automatically shift.

But it doesn't work that way: Lasting change happens when it comes from the inside. When you discover the answer of what's true for you, no one and nothing can take it away from you.

It wasn't until I got pregnant with my son at 36 years old that I made a demand to change this personally destructive and tumultuous cycle with myself and my body. I stopped looking outside myself for an answer or solution and I found true happiness and began to create a life I had always dreamed of.

I know to my core what it's like to have absolutely no self-esteem. I believed I was fat and ugly. It wasn't just the money that I spent searching for an answer and a solution, but it was the 20 years of lost time, lost connections, missing out on weddings, dinner parties, dates, and so much more that almost ruined me!

Looking at me, you might not understand why I wrote this book, but as the saying goes: you can't judge a book by its cover. I wrote this book because I had no idea how much my secret obsession distracted me from LIVING. I spent close to 24 hours a day judging myself, feeling insecure, doubting my beauty, hiding my gifts, and all of my time trying to find a solution to a problem I didn't actually have. It wasn't until I started using the tools and processes in this book that I began to create a life of my dreams. I wrote this book because I realized how many women on the planet spend their entire lives obsessed about changing their bodies and that takes them out of living. The body is not a problem to solve, it is something you should ENJOY living in to CREATE your life!

Growing up, I was a 4-time varsity letter soccer player, a state-qualifying downhill skier, and a really good volleyball player (I was the only sophomore on the Varsity Team). I was good at any sport I tried (except golf - my mother on the other hand is an amazing golfer and is in the Wisconsin Golf Hall of Fame). When I wasn't participating in sports, I was running, biking, playing, swimming, climbing, canoeing, and so much more.

I ate whatever I wanted whenever I wanted and I never worried about food or the impact food would have on my body. I was either active or eating. My Irish Catholic Aunts used to point a finger at me every time they saw me eating (while they causally sipped their wine and smoked their cigarettes) and say:

"Someday all of that is going to go to your thighs".

I used to think they were crazy, but right after I turned 15, I started to feel extremely insecure about my weight, even when there was no logical explanation for my insecurities (I was 6% body fat, weighed 126 pounds, and wore a size 4).

Despite my petite compact muscular frame, I was always on a mission to change my body. I thought that if I could feel better about my body and I could just fit myself into this unrealistic ideal I had, then life would be fine.

I started to diet, restrict, pinch, hide, compare, and obsess. I yo-yo dieted for over 20 years and lost and gained somewhere between 1200 - 1500 pounds (an average of 60 pounds per year for 20 years…some years I lost and gained over 100+ pounds). I spent so much money trying to find the next quick fix that I lost years of my life obsessing over my thighs. I skipped weddings, canceled dates, hid in my house, missed parties, would lie about why I couldn't attend gatherings, I wore a hoodie in disguise at the grocery store, would sneak food and then would stay up until 3am working out in my room hoping I could hide the evidence of my secret late-night bingeing episodes. But behind my giant smile, I had spent most of my adult life secretly feeling miserable, hating myself, trying to hide the pain of how I felt inside, and a lot of times just wishing I wasn't here.

When I looked in the mirror, I didn't see a bright, beautiful, strong, athletic, confident being. Instead, all I could see was a distorted version of my body heavily wrapped in judgments that rattled through me like an unstoppable freight train. When I looked in the mirror all I could see was fat and ugly. This kept me from living my best life, but most of all, it kept me from the happiness that was sitting right in front of me.

I knew at a very young age there was something different about me. I was intuitive and could see things and hear things and know things before they happened. It freaked most people out, especially my Irish Catholic Family, so much so, that at 13, my mother thought it would be a good idea to put me in therapy permanently. My psychiatrist put me on meds shortly after that and was always telling me I was wrong for something. Thus began the downward spiral of thinking I had a problem. If my therapist (the expert) was telling me something was wrong with me, then she must be right and I must be wrong.

Intrinsically, I knew somewhere underneath the wrongness she projected at me, it was simply because I didn't fit the mold of a normal kid. I mean, let's be honest, who is normal?

Not only was I hyper-aware of everyone's thoughts, feelings, and emotions, but I could feel all the judgments people had. At the time, I didn't realize how aware I was, so I started to think that everything I was feeling was mine. For those of you who are intuitive, sensitive, and aware, 98% of everything you think and feel isn't yours! You are just aware of everyone and everything around you, but if you don't acknowledge that, you will think all those crazy thoughts, feelings, emotions, and judgments are yours. And like me, you might be wearing it like an invisible fat suit, never quite able to rid yourself of the heaviness you feel inside.

Because I didn't have this information as a kid, I made myself sick, depressed, and insane with all those crazy judgments. My childhood was a plethora of joy and confusion, laughter and pain, and a constant dichotomy of opposing experiences I always struggled to make sense of. The truth is, it wasn't until I started to write this book that I uncovered some essential components to my story that helped explain why I struggled so deeply with weight issues, body dysmorphia, and an overall sense of hatred for my body. I started to understand all the hidden, underneath the surface causes as to why someone like me might spend their whole life obsessing about their body and not be able to create the change they truly desire.

I lost over 20 years of my life and spent well over $250,000 trying to change my body. Going on a diet seems simple: just change the way you eat. But what most diets don't ever take into consideration are all the underlying psychological components that cause someone to start to think they need to change their body in the first place. I always say: you'll never hear an elephant complain about the size of its ass. And an elephant eats grass all day long. So clearly, it isn't about the food.

It isn't about what you're eating, but rather how you feel that determines how your body will respond to what you're eating. This may seem counterintuitive and against mainstream advice, but most of the time it has nothing to do with WHAT you're eating, but how you feel about yourself WHEN you're eating. I had no idea how deeply trauma can impact the body's ability to be healthy.

Because I was so insecure about my body without ever really having a reason or understanding how much my childhood trauma impacted my body, I went on a mission to find the answers. I was always obsessively seeking something that would take away this pain I never thought I could change. I thought the pain would go away when the weight went away, but in my early 20s I woke up in a hospital weighing 96 pounds and the depression I was feeing was at an all time high, covering me from head to toe. From past life regressions to soul retrievals, to retreats in the jungles with Shamans, from religion to spirituality to meditation, to yoga, dance, dance movement therapy, hypnotherapy, body talk, alternative modalities, energy medicine, and so much more, I spent 20 years traveling around the world, trying anything and everything I could find to discover myself. I even went to Grad School to get my Master's Degree in Somatic Psychology so I could once and for all, uncover the secrets to this mind-body obsession.

No matter how much I uncovered, I always felt like I was missing something. Understanding my past and healing from my pains shouldn't have to be this hard and take this much effort.

After grad school, I came across the tools of Access Consciousness®, and things started to make sense. It was like everything I'd always known, but didn't know I knew was presented in this magical way. I felt a huge sigh of relief. While I was in grad school, I started to get extremely depressed, I started gaining a lot of weight and it felt like my life was getting progressively harder and heavier. I went to grad school so that things could get easier, but that wasn't the case. The more we talked about our problems, the harder it was to change them. It wasn't until I discovered the tools of Access Consciousness and this new approach to life and living that I realized how much we have been taught to talk about our problems as if that is the way to resolve them. But it just isn't true.

The more you talk about your problems, the harder it is to change them. As Einstein says, you cannot solve your problems in the same way you created them. When I stopped talking about my problems, things got easier, not harder. I discovered through this process that problems were a lie. I stopped seeing my challenges as problems, but rather as possibilities disguised as self-imposed obstacles. I started to live in the now and look to the future, rather than the past, for a different possibility.

I learned that I didn't have to follow a structure or someone else's protocol of what they decided was best for me. I learned that asking questions allowed me to discover what was true for me, while conclusions created a solid reality that was dense, unmoveable, heavy, and hard to change. Most of us have been trained to come to conclusions so we can fix what we think is wrong. But think about it … does it ever work?

My conclusion after 20 years of secretly living with the pain of hating myself and my body was that something was wrong with me, I would never be enough, and my body would be a lifelong struggle where I would starve, binge, overeat, berate, shame, belittle, and ultimately abuse it til death do us part.

I remember one day sitting amongst a crowd of people at an introductory evening workshop, listening to this woman talk about the body and sharing her perspective that you can change absolutely anything. In my head, with crossed arms, all up in a huff, I thought to myself as this 110-pound petite blonde who was way too freaking cheery for my unpleasant disposition…

"You don't know my story".

The resentful teenager inside of me who felt slighted by my dysfunctional upbringing decided to give up hanging onto the resentment, anger, and bitterness. Something inside of me saw a glimmer of hope.

So with a suspicious disposition, I started to ask questions to see if there was anything to what she was offering. At this point, I was desperate to change. And frankly, I was sick and tired of hearing myself constantly talk trash to myself. I was sick of trying to change my body. I was sick and tired of waking up feeling like a pathetic fat failure. I was sick of judging myself, feeling insecure, and hanging onto this overall feeling of never being good enough.

What happened next changed my life and is the reason for this book. I started recognizing how many conclusions I had! It was insane. So I started asking questions and they began to open up a space, a curiosity, and a sense of peace that was invigorating. Most of us spend our entire lives trying to come to conclusions about what we think is wrong so we can fix all the things we secretly think are wrong, but it doesn't actually work.

What opened up the door to healing, letting go of wrongness, and truly discovering the world of possibilities available, was this determination to discover what I knew that I didn't know I knew. We need to learn—

to know—that there is nothing wrong with us. There is nothing wrong with our bodies. We just need to stop judging ourselves, and the world around us.

Consciousness includes everything and judges nothing.

Each of you knows something that no one else on the planet knows. And it is up to you to bring what you know, be what you know, and create what you know. The answers you are looking for are inside.

No one else can do it for you. You have within you all the resources available to bring what you know to fruition. If you are willing to trust your inner knowing, over time, with practice, repetition, rest, and determination, you can begin living a life of no judgment. It's a choice (something that we aren't taught).

Judgment is a choice. No judgment is also a choice.

When I discovered judgment was just a choice, it literally changed my entire world. It was like a lightbulb moment that truly transformed not only the way I saw the world, but it transformed the relationship I had with my body, and in turn, it changed my relationship with myself. It was the change I had always been seeking, but never quite knew how to get to.

I let go of hating my body and living a secret life of a love/hate relationship with myself and food, and I began to LIVE!

May you find within the pages of this book a guide full of knowledge, humor, stories, and possibilities to empower you to discover how you can change your mind, change your body, and change your life.

This book and the tools and tips and stories inside will empower you to change the things you think you cannot change. The tools come from my life experience, my voracious desire to study anything that improves human development; Shamanism, Somatic Psychology, Meditation, Access Consciousness, and Energy Medicine. I am not a doctor. I am just obsessed with the human condition and how we can improve ourselves through the power of thought, and perseverance. I spent most of my life hating my body, hiding it, judging it, starving it, obsessively exercising it, picking it apart, ridiculing it, ignoring it, stuffing it, abusing it, and torturing it. I had no idea that the answer to changing it was already inside of me. No one else had the answer but me.

And once I found the answer, I found myself. I restored my self-esteem and I started to see all the amazing possibilities available. It changed my entire life.

Maybe, like me, you have spent much of your life judging your body. Maybe, like me, you thought you would never be able to live without judgment of your body. Maybe, like me, you are far more awake and aware than you had been willing to acknowledge. This book will give you tools to change the things you thought you couldn't change. Then you can begin to see that almost anything is possible. I have seen people lose weight without dieting. I have seen bodies transform with ease. I have seen people get sexier, more radiant, and more alive. I have seen faces get happier and look 10 years younger. I have seen people's spines go from crooked to near straight. I have watched people change their irreversible diseases, change the appearance of their skin, lose over 60 pounds, drop 8 dress sizes, improve their confidence, grow taller, save their marriages, change their relationships, start businesses, take risks, be bold, find happiness, and let go of the things that kept them stuck. I have witnessed so many people create the life they truly desire, overcome obstacles with so much ease, create miracles, and so much more.

Most people would call it a miracle. What I know is when you talk to the body and actually listen without judgment and without a point of view, anything can change.

What could you change if you stopped judging you?

Want to find out?

*** The truth is this book isn't just about the body, this book is an invitation to tap into your knowing, to trust your gut, to become the expert of your own body, and your own reality. The truth is this book is the beginning of you expressing your truth, paying attention to the unseen so that instead of distracting yourself with your problems, you actually create your life by paying attention to the whispers of possibilities. They are always all around you. When you pay attention to them, your life can grow...

Introduction

"The World Doesn't Need More Diets.
The World Needs to Love the Skin They Are In."
—*Katherine McIntosh*

Do you love going on a diet? If you're like most people the word *diet* probably doesn't make you happy. You might even have a long dieting history to go along with it. Think about it. Does the idea of a *diet* make you happy?

Perhaps the idea of having a body you LOVE makes you happy. But the truth is, the majority of the world—from supermodels to actors, moms to musicians, dads to artists, lawyers to doctors, teenagers to children are not happy with something about their physical appearance. If you asked the 7 billion people on the planet today if they would change something about their bodies, it would be a rare occurrence for someone to say they wouldn't change anything.

In a world where judgment is accepted as a way of being in the world, so many people are searching for something to make them happy. We have created a society that is result orientated. But what if we became a society that seeks happiness as the true result of living?

Instead of looking for a result to lose 10 pounds, what if the real result, you were seeking, was to be happy? What if we were a society that learned to celebrate ourselves instead of criticizing ourselves? The purpose of a diet is to lose weight. But how many people are actually successful on a diet long term?

The truth is, that most diets are not sustainable. They do not promote a lifestyle that generates living, but rather, the sheer nature of a diet is to promote dying, lack, restriction, and judgment as a source for change. That's pretty backwards if you ask me. Have you ever gone on a diet and a few days in felt like you were dying of hunger?

When was the last time you were truly happy on a diet?

You might have been happy with the results, but the problem with most diets is that they are driven by imposing rules on you. These include restrictions, time calculations, calorie counting, food measuring, and, most of all, JUDGMENT. You cannot be aware of what's true for you when you are judging you.

Judgment and awareness cannot exist simultaneously. So if you are constantly judging whether or not you are doing something right to get a result, but you aren't focused on being happy and acknowledging whether that action brings you long term joy, then how are you supposed to be aware of what would actually work for you?

Let's be clear. I am not talking about short term happiness, but long term happiness based on what would actually make you happy. If changing your body and getting healthier and paying more attention to your nutrition, exercise, and overall choices would make you happy, then it's about long term happiness.

For example, a piece of cake in a moment might make you sooooooo happy, but if you repeat eating a piece of cake everyday, the long term effects will most likely sabotage your happiness. This is about JOY. Long-term.

> *"Joy is only possible when you embrace how imperfect you are and actually love it."*
> —*Dr. Dain Heer*

Diets paint this picture that if you follow the directions and restrict yourself, you will get the results and you will be happy. But how many people do you know for whom that has actually worked long-term?

The problem is that diets are an action outside of the ordinary. Please know, I am not against diets, I am just not in favor of teaching people that they need to cut off their awareness of their body in order to achieve the change they are looking for. I know true change is possible for anyone, but it has to start with a shift in perspective, a mindset diet, and then the actions that follow can create lasting change, but action absent of the mindset to back it up will never create lasting change.

In order for you to have true lasting happiness with your body and life, I believe there are a few special ingredients required when you approach any action related to your body.

One: It needs to be something that you adapt as a part of your lifestyle, not just something you choose temporarily. It has to become a part of you.

Two: It has to make you happy enough to invest your time, energy, and resources long-term.

Three: It has to be a commitment to long-term living, not short-term instant gratification.

The problem with most diets is that they promise results as long as you follow a protocol, but that protocol rarely integrates easily into someone's lifestyle. It usually involves restricting, cutting, and sacrificing. The diet sets up an unrealistic expectation that the only way to achieve desired results is if you starve, restrict, and sacrifice. That is not long-term living.

Have you ever seen a business grow almost overnight, only to have it crash and burn just as quickly as it developed? That kind of business model is rarely sustainable over time. It's the businesses that build off of, and are driven by, the sheer love of it that actually succeed. These businesses develop, grow, and flourish over time. There is a foundation from which to build, scale, and grow.

> *"Life needs to be more than just solving everyday problems. You need to wake up and be excited about the future."*—*Elon Musk*

Your body is not a problem to be solved. If that is your sole purpose, you will miss out on living. Sadly, I know this from experience. I cannot tell you the number of times I missed events, weddings, connecting with friends, following through on all of those insane business ideas, laughing, playing, creating, and future-building all because I was so consumed by how I looked and wished I was thinner.

I wasted an incredible amount of time researching the next fad diet that promised to deliver the results. Yet it was always under the guise of promising to myself...

This time, it will be different. This time, I will follow through. This time...

Unfortunately, for me, there was always a next time...to the tune of tens of thousands, and then hundreds of thousands, of dollars spent trying to fix myself. I learned the hard and expensive way, that it didn't work. I know I'm not alone. The average American woman will spend over 30 years of her life on a diet, will go on an average of 8 diets a year, and will spend an average of $1,422 a year on diets. Over 30 years, that's over $42,000.

On diets.

And that's just on diets. It doesn't include money spent on gym memberships, yoga studios, personal trainers, beauty products, exercise gimmicks, teas, collagen, and who knows what else. We are talking about $1,422 a year on good ol' diets. Calorie counting, food restricting, protein measuring *diets*.

Fortunately, the world is changing and people are waking up and finding ways to incorporate individual needs. Traditional diets do not take into consideration the individual's lifestyle habits, desires, dreams, aspirations, and already built-in food choices.

Traditional diets just deliver a regimented protocol. But losing weight, if it's going to last long-term, cannot be a military, boot camp experience. Losing weight, changing shape, transforming one's health needs to consider individual desires as much more important than the act of shedding a few pounds. Whenever I personally declared it was time to lose weight, I almost always gained more weight, craved more foods, and had a hard time stopping when I was full…

The purpose of losing weight was because I always wanted to feel better about myself. The comical thing is: no diet ever really made me feel better about myself. I usually found myself criticizing, judging, pinching, skimping, and ridiculing myself more. What I've discovered through my own personal journey is that choosing to love the skin you are in, to acknowledge and appreciate the body as it is, that is when true change (both inside and out) can occur.

After all, aren't we all just trying to feel beautiful and be the best version of ourselves we can be? We won't get there by judging ourselves or comparing ourselves to other people. We won't get there if we don't develop a healthy relationship with our own bodies.

Beauty is a unique experience for everyone. And everyone is beautiful in their own way, but studies show that most people don't believe they are. When I came across the following statistic, I was shocked and it made me look at this even deeper:

Only 4% of women all over the world consider themselves beautiful…

My desire for this book is to change that percentage. I want to contribute to you exploring how you can get out of what locks you into judgment so that you can see that you are beautiful and that your body *is* just right for you.

Can you imagine an elephant complaining about the size of it's ass? No!

That would be absolutely insane! Just like an elephant, or a giraffe, or a lion, there is nothing wrong with you and there never was. You are just different and unique and you cannot compare yourself to anyone else. So strut your stuff and celebrate your unique-ness.

It is okay to want to change, but the change has to be navigated from a completely different vantage point. Judgment does not create happiness. Change needs to come from within, from getting uncomfortable creating a relationship and a reality with your body you've never had before.

It may be uncomfortable at first, but if you stick with it, you will find a level of freedom and joy that won't only change your body, it will change your business, your relationships, your financial reality, and your life. Would that bring you joy?

If you truly desire to change, then you have all the resources inside of you to make that change. The only reason we don't change is because we create excuses as to why we can't achieve something when, in reality, without knowing it, we are scared of our own brilliance.

> *"Our deepest fear is not that we are inadequate. Our deepest fear is that we are powerful beyond measure. It is our light, not our darkness, that most frightens us. We ask ourselves, 'Who am I to be brilliant, gorgeous, talented, fabulous?' Actually, who are you not to be?"*
> *—Marianne Williamson*

To those bold enough to begin the journey towards no judgment, keep going and don't give up. This is *your* journey! And your brilliance may just surprise you. When you stop shying away from that which makes you different, you will create a completely different reality with all the things you thought were wrong with you. You will discover those were the things that were the strongest about you.

Why write a book on dieting?

At the age of 15, in total despair and misery at a whopping 126lbs and very fit and muscular, I went on my first diet. It was the first of close to 200 different diets and over $250,000 spent on gadgets, videos, books, classes, teas, workshops, therapy, and so much more—all desperate attempts to change what I felt I needed to fix. It took me over 20 years to discover that there was no external solution to the fact that I was dying on the inside. What needed to be changed was that I needed to see myself as beautiful from the inside out.

It isn't that the diet is the problem….

It's that only 4% of women worldwide consider themselves beautiful. The epidemic is thinking we need to fix something instead of embracing that every single one of us is beautiful.

Since the age of 15, I have tried Jenny Craig, Nutri-System, Weight Watchers, shakes, laxatives, not eating, starvation diets, the grapefruit diet, the thigh master, the sit up cruncher, bow flex, grapefruit seed extract, goji berries, green tea extract, tulsi tea, keto, dancing in the jungles of South America, soul retrievals, past life regressions, lean protein, power walking, mountain climbing, mountain biking, dancing, breathing, meditating, acupuncture, massage, eating veggies only…anything that had a promise of weight loss. Anything that had the word diet in it I've either tried or mulled it over for days, or weeks, or months, or years as to whether *that* would be the one thing that would finally take me out of my misery.

I've tried the master cleanse, the Atkins diet, the 15 minutes a day diet, the South Beach diet, the paleo diet, the listening to your intuition diet, and some fit/fat diet that promised to reduce the fat on my body by 30% (like most, it worked temporarily). I've taken every supplement under the sun. I've done a 10 day transformation cleanse. I even considered liposuction before going on a date, when I was 20, because I was horrified by the shape of my thighs. At the time, if there was a chance I was going to be seen in shorts, or a fitting dress, or a swimsuit, I would think of everything I possibly could do to either hide my body or find a way to change it. If there was a possibility that something would change my body, I did it.

I've tried to yoga weight off and I've done every Beach Body program they've ever made. I've tried to drink my weight off; I've tried to smoke and Diet Coke my weight off. I've gone days without eating, weeks of only juicing. My efforts resulted in serious health problems: I became anorexic and bulimic. I've been to Overeaters Anonymous, eating disorder groups, outpatient therapy groups, and one-on-one therapy. I've been put on Prozac, mood disorder medications, and a million other things. I tried hypnotizing myself to stop the insane starvation/overeating cycle.

None of them changed the one thing that needed to change. I needed to **STOP** thinking that something was wrong with me or my body. You see, the problem isn't diets.

The problem is that we think there is something wrong with our bodies.

This book is not about permission to eat McDonald's every day and blame me. I am not a doctor or certified psychologist, and there is no medical advice in this book. My only hope is the drive for you to push yourself to discover what is true for you. No one knows more about you than you. And no one can tell you what's true for you other than you.

My experience is that things last for long periods of time *only* if we are invested emotionally in the process as much as we are invested in the outcome. **If you don't love the process of getting yourself there, it will never last.**

While I am not a licensed psychologist, I am obsessed with exploring the psychology of the body and mind. For over 20 years I have been a seeker, diving into energy medicine, Shamanism, energy work, alternative therapies and energy modalities, spent a year in a Master's Somatic Psychology Program — and any modality that addresses both the physical and mental aspects of thoughts, feelings, and emotions.

For 20 years I was constantly seeking, searching, uncovering, and trying to discover the truths that were never explained to me. My whole life I have been obsessed with the unseen mysteries of things that could almost never be explained. From blindfold ritual dancing, soul retrievals, past life regressions, spirit animals, ancestral lineage dances, ecstatic movement, alternative therapies, sound baths, native american sweat lodges, hypnotism, and everything else you can think of.

All of them made a huge impact, but it wasn't until I discovered some of the tools of Access Consciousness® where I was actually able to completely change the one thing I thought I couldn't: my body. This book is a compilation of everything I've ever studied, thought, experimented with, and uncovered. From the tools of Access, to the studies of Shamanism, to Dance Movement Therapy, to all the healing modalities I ever learned, studied, and self-taught, this book has pieces of me in all of it.

Studying and being curious about everything allowed me to incorporate individuality into how I think about lifestyle changes related to the body. Because the truth is that a diet is just one person's success story. What may work for one person may not work for another. In order to work, it has to be intuitive and make sense to each person; it must fulfill their needs as well as invite the person's character & lifestyle needs into the process. But I think the biggest discovery is that it has to address everything underneath the surface. Change isn't just about action. Change needs to incorporate the underbelly of the subconscious and shed light on all the dark places.

> *"Knowing is not enough; we must apply. Willing is not enough; we must do."* —Bruce Lee

This book is intended to encourage you to change the way you see yourself. It is intended to encourage you to become your own ally...so that, maybe one day, when your boyfriend, girlfriend, husband, wife, lover, or friend compliments you, your body, your butt, or the size of your thighs, you may actually believe them and receive the compliment.

This book isn't about dieting. While it speaks to body image and self-esteem, it comes from a different way of looking at everything. This book is about the judgments we have and the ideas of beauty we've been taught. And it challenges you to question everything. I am not against diets, I am just against giving up your awareness in favor of someone else's promise that you'll get results. The only way to get results long term is to develop a relationship with yourself and with your body that empowers you to know.

When you stop following everyone else's advice, thinking you'll get results and you stop judging what you eat, what your body looks like, what clothes you wear, what size you are, how much you think you need to exercise and how much you haven't exercised, you begin to have a sense of what is available to create in and with a body that feels good.

You are the expert of your body. No one else. So educate yourself, empower yourself, experiment with what might work, and let go of the things that don't work. This isn't a one-size-fits-all experiment. This is a unique and catered experience where you take your body with you.

Once you stop judging yourself you can function from a place where anything is possible. This applies to any area of your life where you judge yourself.

This book will ask you to set aside everything you've been taught and believe about the body, food, and weight, and open up to the possibility of discovering a whole new way of living. Here you will find tools and questions that will help you listen to your body to create a relationship with it you may have never thought possible.

From someone who never thought it would be possible, it is. There is freedom and when you find it, it will change your entire life! And when you get what actually works for you, no one can take that away from you. Please don't believe everything I say. The point of this book is for you to begin to question what will work for you. To find your truth. And to find the brilliance you've always been. You got this! Your time is now!

Chapter 1
My Closet Nightmare

"As long as you are doing judgment instead of choice, nothing will ever change."
—*Gary Douglas*

Judgments and Your Body - Masking the Judgments We Hide from Ourselves

There I was in the middle of my closet, curled up in a fetal position on top of a giant pile of clothes. Tears streamed down my face, my hands were sweaty, and I was breathing hard. The heat coming off of my body was palpable from all the panting. I was shaky, my heart beating out of my chest.

How could this have happened!?

In a panic, I looked up at all the empty hangers and realized I had tried on almost every outfit I owned in an attempt to find the perfect one that would make me feel sexy, alive, and confident. Clearly, given my panicked state, I had failed miserably. And when I looked at the clock I realized I was late for an extremely important event where my significant other was the star of the show. I had just wasted two hours of my life in a hell hole of judgment, shame, criticism, and not enough. I had spent two hours deep in judgment of my body, and now I was a miserable mess.

How could this be? How could I have gotten so sucked in that I lost track of time? How is it possible that I couldn't find anything to wear? What was wrong with me? Just like my closet, it felt like all my emotions were piled on the floor. I was a hot mess of tears and screams and vacant, empty, dissatisfied promises to myself.

That was my wake up call.

Because there wasn't an outfit in the world that could have fixed how I felt about myself on the inside. Nothing could take away the pain of self-judgment that had plagued my existence since I was a teen. The truth was, I hated myself. What's more, I hated how I felt about my body, and it didn't matter if I was 96 pounds or 160 pounds. I had an ache in the pit of my stomach that was constantly telling me I wasn't enough. I wanted to rip it out.

In college, I went on this crazed quest to see how little I could eat, how far I could run, how many mountains I could climb, how many Diet Cokes I could pound, how many cigarettes I could smoke, how little I could weigh. I was the picture-perfect poster child for anorexia. Simultaneously, I was in complete denial. At 96 pounds, I almost died.

But it wasn't until my brother's high school graduation from military academy that I realized something was really wrong. I was standing right on the edge of where the graduates would walk, ready to surprise my brother after not seeing him for 5 months. Everyone was hugging their loved ones, greeted with ear-to-ear smiles full of pride. And then it came time for me to give my brother a congratulatory hug, and as I smiled with open arms, he walked right by me.

My heart sank. I realized that I had gotten so skinny, I was unrecognizable. An emaciated skeleton, my own brother didn't even recognize me! Maybe the most depressing part of this situation was that I still saw myself as fat and ugly. No amount of dieting, starving, exercising, or hiding underneath my baggy clothes could make me feel beautiful.

I spent years thinking that if I could get my body down to the size, weight, and shape I had decided was an acceptable ideal, then I would be happy. But the truth was, no matter what I did to change the outside to feel beautiful, I had too many judgments inside. So it didn't matter what I did, I still felt numb to the pain of never feeling good enough. It wasn't until much later in life that I realized the judgments hadn't changed and that is what I needed to address. So often it's the energy unerneath the situation that needs to be addressed. If someone cuts themselves deeply, you can't just address the bleeding, you have to address what's underneath the bleeding to stop it.

> *"Girls see enough of this body we can't imitate, that we'll never be able to obtain... these unrealistic expectations. It's better to look healthy and strong." —Jennifer Lawrence*

You cannot judge yourself into beauty. Have you ever tried it?

Diets are designed to fuel judgment.

The diet industry feeds off of the idea that if you judge you—it means you have to cut off your awareness—then you will spend money trying to solve the problem you've decided is real. The entire industry feeds off of your insecurities. It thrives on the bet that you won't feel empowered when it comes to losing weight and getting fit. So it offers a million different options, with a million different messages of how to lose weight. Remember that the average American woman in search of losing weight will try up to 8 diets a year. If you try 8 different diets, it's likely that all 8 of those did not lead to the peace and happiness you were looking for.

So now, if you're the average American woman, you've spent up to $1,422 in the year and will be on and off diets for 30 years. To reiterate how insane the spending becomes, that means spending over $42,660 on diets, on average, in one woman's lifetime. (Good thing I'm above average and have squandered over $250,000 trying to fix my body.)

But the truth is that our bodies do not need fixing.

The idea that your body needs fixing is a flawed premise. The diet industry as a whole is not here to educate you, inspire you, or encourage you. Some diets do promote self-awareness. Up until recently, most of the diet industry wasn't interested in empowering you to know that you know. The more confused you feel, the more money you'll spend. The diet industry hopes you will feel powerless and dependent on external sources outside of yourself. The less empowered you feel on the inside, the more money you will give to people who claim to be experts in their fields of health, fitness, and weight loss. They might be experts in the sense that what they're selling worked for some people, but it doesn't mean it will work for you—especially if your weight, body image, and self-esteem is connected to your emotions.

Do Diets Work?

YES. Diets work when you use a diet to intuitively understand what does and doesn't work for you. Diets also work temporarily as long as you cut off your awareness, starve yourself, and go against what feels natural and intuitive. I am not anti-diet. I am against trying to change your body by cutting off your awareness.

So you try a diet in hopes it will deliver the results you crave and give you the answers you've spent your whole life searching for. But when that fails, instead of walking away from bad advice, you dive into another diet or health regiment. And before you know it, you become obsessed with the idea that there has to be something out there that will work for your body (or worse… you secretly feel like something is wrong with you and your body).

The key to a diet isn't a diet at all. It's about developing a healthy relationship with your body and learning to listen to your body's needs and wishes. Think about how relationships take time to grow and develop. It takes time to trust your heart and surrender the walls of protection that only serve to separate you.

In 2019, the diet industry grossed $72 billion. Clearly, the industry is not interested in you knowing what you know about your body, without judgment, because it would lose money. The industry depends on you judging your body. The more you judge you, the more time you'll spend trying to find a solution, and the more money you'll be willing to spend on things that promise to help you change your body.

How many times have you tried a diet only to realize that it doesn't really work for you? The way diets are created are not designed to make you feel empowered. They want you to empower a source outside of yourself. The fact is, most diets just fuel your insecurities, reinforcing ideas like: you don't have enough willpower, you're big boned, you have a slow metabolism, you are weak, you're not dedicated, your thyroid is off...etcetera, etcetera, etcetera.

Up until recently, the vital thing that's missing from the diet industry is the willingness to empower you to develop a healthy relationship with your body. Diets want you to follow a formula, but there is no formula out there for relationships. And one of the most important relationships you'll ever have is the one you have with your body.

Your body may not speak English (or French, Spanish, or Portuguese), but your body does speak in energy. It's clear as day if you're willing to listen. The trick is to become aware of all the different ways in which your body communicates with you.

Would you be happy if you stayed in a committed relationship long-term if there wasn't good communication? What if all you received from your partner was a constant barrage of ridicule and judgment as to what you're doing wrong and why you aren't good enough?

Most people would not stay. And if they did stay, they would likely be unhappy. When you stop listening to your body, when you bark orders at it, when you ridicule, judge, and belittle it—you are creating a toxic relationship with your body and expecting it not to fight back.

But the body *does* fight back. It wakes up and it starts to create some form of pain, discomfort, or disease until you begin to pay attention to it. Obesity, for example, is a disease. The body gains weight, not because of food, but because of judgment. Wrinkles develop prematurely. The skin starts to break down, bones start to ache, joints hurt—everything starts to talk back. Some people blame their bodies' rapid decline of pain, weight gain, disease or wrinkles on getting older, but personally I don't think it has anything to do with age. I think it has to do with judgment.

When you judge yourself, it creates a discord. Going back to the analogy of a relationship, if the person you are in a relationship with starts getting upset with you, or judging you, or cutting you down, or barking orders at you, it's much more difficult to want to do something nice for them in the moment. Hence why it's hard to change something if you are judging it. On the other hand, if your relationship is grateful for you, just as you are, it's much easier to do something that contributes to them. It's also easier to change a behavior. When you have gratitude for your body, it is much easier to change those things you think you cannot change.

Gratitude is a very different vibration compared to judgment. In fact gratitude is one of the highest forms of vibration on the planet. It is even higher than love because love has so many definitions based on one's experience of love, whereas gratitude is universal.

> *"If you do what is easy, your life will be hard. If you do what is hard, your life will be easy."*
> *—Les Brown*

My philosophy is, the more you judge you, the harder life gets. The less you judge you, the easier life gets. It's a pretty simple formula that I believe can withstand the test of time. From most people's perspectives, it is hard to go against the grain, to listen to your knowing, to feel like you don't fit, so we go the easy route…

A diet, a quick fix, thinking something is wrong. But the truth is that is not the easy way…nor is it the effective way.

Have you ever been in a relationship where you constantly felt like you were being judged?

Now, let's imagine how you would feel if every person you were in a relationship with told you how grateful they are for you, how amazing, beautiful, sexy, and strong you are? Would that create a different future? When you are grateful for your body, what does that create? When you judge your body, when you belittle it, what does that create?

Take a moment to think about it: How much judgment do you have of your body, your food choices, and your exercise routine when you decide you need to lose weight? Be honest.

I don't know about you, but everytime I tell myself I need to lose weight all I want to do is eat more. I crave sugar; I dream about croissants, donuts, cake, and pizza. As I dream about those things—while simultaneously subconsciously telling myself that I can't have those things—it creates a polarity in my body. That polarity creates a tug of war; it upsets the homeostasis flow in the body and activates an internal fight-or-flight response. When we are in this survival mode, the adrenaline pump in the body increases and it is very difficult to relax, which means the body is never allowed to truly rest and relax.

Rest is essential. Relieving the stress responses from the body allows the body to transform with ease. Most people ask the body to lose weight. I don't know about you, but asking that of my body never makes me feel excited. Instead of feeling excited and inspired, I put pressure on myself. I end up criticizing all my choices and in turn, I usually end up gaining weight.

Judgments are heavy. They weigh a ton, and they kill our bodies.

Judgments are solid and dense, and judgment and awareness cannot exist simultaneously. Would you rather create your life through judgment or through the awareness you gain from listening to what your body is telling you?

When you start following the awareness of what your body desires, you can begin to create a totally different relationship with your body. That is where the magic is.

Learning to love the skin you are in—no matter what size, shape, or skin color you have—releases the judgments locked up in your body that limit every area of your life.

This is an exploration of going on a different kind of diet with your body, one that removes judgments and adds joy...

Remember, this is about **BEING HAPPY.**

This is a roadtrip to awareness. With awareness, everything is available to you. Are you tired of making yourself wrong? Are you done wasting your life finding fault with your body?

Is it time for a different journey? To enjoy living and be happy?

This book is designed to open you up to love the skin you're in and create the life of your dreams. To have more ease, more joy, and more fun. Shouldn't the purpose of life be to have fun? Because when you laugh, you change the planet; you heal your body, and you heal the earth.

Anger and judgment do the opposite: they destroy your body and destroy the earth. What would your life be like if you had more self-esteem, more peace of mind and greater awareness? What would your life be like if you woke up happy?

Most people go on diets because, ultimately, they want to FEEL happy.

Yet most diets make you feel more depressed and more disconnected from you. Most diets make you feel some combination of hungry, achy, irritable, intense, and angry. Years ago I was in New York City and met up with a friend I hadn't seen in several months. She looked amazing, but as we approached each other for a big hug I could see she was hiding something.

"You look amazing!" I said.

Tears started streaming down her face. She tried holding back the tears but couldn't. Even though she had lost 40 pounds, the ache inside of her was palpable. "I feel awful," she said. "I thought losing weight would make me happy, but I realize that no amount of dieting is going to fix the things I've been hiding underneath the weight. I feel so depressed and I realize I have a lot of emotional work I need to do. I think I need your program."

When she said that, she was referring to an online course, The No Judgment Diet. It's a course that invites you to discover what you know. You are the source, the catalyst, and the change. You have everything inside of you you need to succeed and to know you have all the wisdom inside of you to make the changes. The challenge is: Are you willing to listen?

You see the body doesn't speak in language, it speaks in energy. And if you have been disconnected from your body, then it's hard to listen. The path is to discover the way your body speaks to you. There are a million ways that it is speaking to you every day. Inside this book is the wisdom to invite you to discover what you know.

The tools in this book won't tell you what to do. It won't tell you where you're right or where you're wrong. It won't give you a formula or tell you not to eat your favorite foods. Instead, these tools will invite you to discover *what you know*. It will help you to discover *what your body knows*. This road trip we're on is about inviting you to feel empowered—to know what you know, even if no one else agrees with you. It doesn't matter what anyone else thinks. It matters how YOU FEEL.

I'm going to be blunt for a minute: please stop allowing outside influences to affect your internal empowered sense of self. No one can tell you how to live your life. No one knows more about your body than you. So stop handing over your power to others.

Quiet the judgments, quiet the mind, and go inside.

What you discover may surprise and delight you. You are an untapped resource, and the world has been waiting for you. When you begin to quiet your judgments and tap into your awareness, you can start to listen to the subtle possibilities where happiness is beckoning you to play. You are not wrong, and you have never been wrong. You are an awake, empowered being. When you begin to function from that place, not only can your body change but your entire life can change,

I have heard this from many people over the years. They say, Katherine, I didn't believe you when you said my whole life could change! You were right! This is amazing!

When your body is communicating, instead of going to the conclusion that the pain or weight in your body is yours, ask a question. Be curious. Investigate and then listen.

Whenever something is occurring inside your body, the first thing you should always ask is: Is this mine?

I have asked so many people if the disease they are carrying, the pain they are having, or the extra weight they are experiencing, is it yours?

The majority of the time, you will realize that what you are feeling, sensing, and perceiving isn't yours.

If it doesn't change by asking that question, or you don't get lighter when you ask it, then continue asking more questions.

For example, if your knees hurt, you can ask: What does your body need? What do you need? What needs do you have that you are ignoring?

If you are having pains in your neck, you can ask: Who or what is a pain in your neck? Are you sticking your neck out for someone or something?

If you are struggling with your weight, and no matter how little you eat, your body keeps gaining weight, you can ask: What is your body waiting for? Who or what are you waiting for? What is weighing you down? What are you waiting to choose? Is now the time to stop waiting? Is your body aware of judgments?

If you are experiencing throat problems or you have been continuously coughing, you can ask: What are you unwilling to say? What is your body trying to cough up? Is something else in your body that isn't yours? What's the lie that's keeping your body at the effect of coughing up what isn't yours?

The body will always tell you the truth energetically but it won't always come in the from of an answer. So you have to practice translating the energy your body is communicating. Just like in a relationship, you have to practice getting to learn your partner's non verbal energetic clues.

When you have conflict in your relationships, the person you're communicating with may say something and you know that their words aren't matching what is actually occurring. So sometimes you have to listen to the energy, not listen to the answer. Most communication is non verbal and the body is no different. It rarely communicates a clear answer, but rather attempts to give you the energy so you can follow your awareness and pay attention to the non verbal cues. When you get it, you'll know.

It starts one day, one moment, one choice at a time. A healthy, vibrant, alive relationship stands the test of time *only* when you are willing to show up for you and be present with who and what is in front of you. When you are willing to lower your barriers and engage in a moment-by-moment experience with it. Over time, you change. So does your body.

People change their minds all the time. Your body is no different. What helped you feel sexy, vibrant, and fit last year may not work this year. Your body may have changed its mind. So be present and pay attention to the subtleties. Go with the flow and change with the changes. Pay attention and you will learn to trust you instead of doubting you.

Chapter 2
Your Reflection Isn't Real

"If you wanna make the world a better place, take a look at yourself, then make that change." —Michael Jackson

When most people look in the mirror, they don't see themselves. They see their judgments.

Shortly after the infamous clothes incident in my closet, I puffed up my chest, gave myself a few hundred mini pep talks, and proclaimed loudly to the world (aka my bathroom mirror) that I was going to, once and for all, get fit no matter what it took!

So I ordered the latest get-fit workout available, and a week later a package arrived at my front door. Like a giddy school girl, I tore it open. As the excitement rushed like waves over my body, I thought to myself, "This is It! This is the answer I have been waiting for."

That scenario was an all-too-familiar pattern that would repeat itself over and over again: I would decide enough was enough, take action, go all in for a day, a week, maybe even a month. But then, inevitably, I wouldn't see the results I wanted. So I would put whatever program or pill I had bought in the closet or on a shelf, sigh a giant, weighted sigh, and then wait until the next lightning strike of inspiration that came with a declaration of "Enough is enough!"

> *"Insanity is doing the same thing over and over again, and expecting different results."*—Albert Einstein

I went on diet after diet after diet and never experienced the results that were promised. I never really got anywhere except feeling worse about myself and having far less money in the bank. Every diet I tried created temporary results, but I could never maintain it. Is it any wonder that "die" is in the word "diet"? They are all about restrictions. So after every short-term diet experience, I would eventually end up with a little more cushion around my waist or thighs, as well as an invisible weight of judgment that quietly eroded my self-esteem.

Insanity is doing diet after diet and expecting something different. A diet is a diet is a diet. No one diet is really any different from any other. I can say from experience that *diets* are the problem. You are not the problem. Your body is not the problem. Our addiction to judgment is the problem. We think that if we cannot solve something we should look to an outside expert for advice.

But the key to happiness cannot be found outside ourselves. The key is self-awareness, trusting yourself, and recognizing that you are the greatest resource for what you know. We just haven't been taught to be our own experts. We haven't been encouraged to slow down enough to know that *we know*.

You *know*. Your body knows. And you've always known.

I wish I would have known what I know now, it probably would have saved me hundreds of thousands of dollars, thousands of hours of heartache, pain, insecurity, and disappointment. It would have saved me from unrealistic expectations every time I spent money on something I wished would work.

So there I was in giddy excitement: the package had finally arrived. The next morning I woke up early, put in the DVD (yes, this was many years ago), and went through its rigorous exercise routine: squats, push ups, crunches, burpees, side planks, and more. I felt empowered, alive, and sexy, all of which reaffirmed my conclusion that I found the answer!

[Note to self: Don't ever come to conclusions.]

I read through the food guidebook and mapped out my meals for the week, all lean protein and veggies. "I can do this!" I thought. The next day, I woke up early again, put on my workout gear, turned on the DVD, and pulled out my weights and yoga mat. I sweat, I swore, I grunted, I cried. I measured my food. I followed the step-by-step guidelines. I wanted to skip days but didn't. I did it all.

After 30 days, I was feeling rather proud of my accomplishments, and I decided to measure my success. I had 60 more days to go. So I went back to my closet with a hop in my step. I couldn't wait to see the improvements.

Well, what happened next was heartbreaking. After almost two hours, I found myself back in the exact same situation as before I started the program. I was slumped over a giant pile of clothes with tears streaming down my face. I felt like I might have a panic attack. I was a complete failure. How could this be?!?!

There is no way I could be BIGGER!!!!

I followed the program, I ate what I was told, I woke up every morning and did the exercises; I sweat, I grunted, I cried, and at the end of each day celebrated my victory, another day of showing up for me.

Yet, at the end of 30 days, none of my clothes fit me and I had an Oscar worthy meltdown on that all too familiar pile of clothes in my closet. You might be wondering: How could none of your clothes fit you? Weren't you wearing what was in your closet?

Well, yes and no. It was summer in Colorado, which was flowy dress weather, so I was pretty much wearing a handful of dresses over and over again. (I was in my early 30s and still reliving parts of my carefree hippie days.) So when I walked into the closet that day, I went back to my skinny jeans and winter clothes, clothes that I used to measure how my body was doing.

That was when disaster struck. The fight-or-flight autonomic response systems took over and I was done for. So after the gut wrenching horror of realizing that no matter how hard I worked, restricted, sweated, and picked apart what I allowed myself to enjoy, it *still* wasn't enough. I walked away from that experience feeling more like a failure than I ever had before.

After 30 days of restriction and hard work, I felt WORSE not better. Don't get me wrong, I am all for hard work and dedicating yourself to making your life better. But to go all-in with blood, sweat, and tears and come out worse than before is just demoralizing. There was a blood curdling surrender inside my bones shouting, "ENOUGH IS ENOUGH!"

I threw my hands up in the air, a full-body surrender, and I decided to do something crazy. If I had just spent 30 days avoiding all the foods I loved and I *gained* weight, I decided to give myself permission to eat the foods I loved and see what happened. The one food that I loved more than any other, but also judged myself while eating more harshly than any other, was ICE CREAM.

I wondered what would happen if I gave myself permission to eat my absolute favorite food for the next 30 days. (I also ate other foods, not ONLY ice cream; I just added it in every day). For 30 straight days I allowed myself to eat ice cream for breakfast or lunch. However, I didn't allow myself to eat ice cream after 3pm. I knew better. Because my past had included compulsive overeating, the control freak in me had to put a stipulation in there so that I wouldn't binge eat, go down a rabbit hole, and just make things worse. I knew myself well enough to know that at that time in my life, considering the fragile state of existence I was in, creating some parameters would serve me well. Guess what happened in those 30 days?

I lost 10 freaking pounds! I couldn't believe it. That experience was a catalyst that helped me begin to see that almost all my fears about food and my body were a lie.

Food does not create your body. Judgments do.

That moment taught me that most people are just guessing what would work for them. Some people have figured it out, but the vast majority don't understand what it takes to create a long-lasting, healthy relationship with their body. It's like this mystery that most people feel they can't solve. But like any relationship, a healthy relationship with your body takes patience, communication, the willingness to listen, and allowance. The only difference between your relationship with your body and your relationship with other people is that your body doesn't speak in words. It speaks in energy.

We need to stop treating ourselves as if we don't have the information. We do. We just have never been taught how to cultivate self-awareness. No one can tell you how to be a good parent; that is your journey between you and your children. No one can tell you how to be CEO of your own company. No one can tell you how to do your intimate relationships. They are all journeys of self-discovery, not prescriptions you take.

I believe self-awareness is the key to peace, fulfillment, and happiness. Stop judging you and nearly all of your worry, fear, and anxiety just goes away. After 30 days of ice cream and realizing I had lost weight, I was fascinated. All mainstream advice would have highly advised against such an atrocity.

When I started traveling and teaching The No Judgment Diet workshops, I met a journalist who was interested in my experience. I told her my ice cream story and the first thing out of her mouth was, "OMG! Did you have your cholesterol checked?" My cholesterol was just fine! My body was happy. I learned that being happy, grateful, alive, and joyful changes your body quicker and faster than any diet program.

After that experience, I had a newfound respect for my body. I discovered that if I ate when I was happy and truly enjoyed what I was eating, it made me happy, I ate less, I played more, and my body started to shift. In stark contrast, when I was critical of what I was eating, when I was obsessed about losing weight or judged what I should or shouldn't eat, then I felt heavy. Even when I ate a salad, the food sat on me like an elephant.

It just isn't about the food.

It's about how you feel, what you think, and whether or not you are being present in the moment and savoring every experience. Drink in the sunsets, eat up the adventure, bask in the joy of laughing with a friend over a delicious meal. Eat cake. Drink wine. Play in the desert. Hike up a mountain. But whatever you do, stop dedicating your waking hours to judgments.

The truth is, when we judge, we stop playing. We stop being curious and we start to take on the weight of everyone's judgments.

Think about how a 5 year old girl is not very likely to say, "Mommy, I don't want to go swimming because I'm afraid of what I look like in a swimsuit." Life is too short. Get over yourself. Your body was designed to PLAY!

When you stop judging what you look like, you have space to create your life. Life is about creating. Imagine if your life started to be about creating the future instead of fixing the past?

"Look yourself in the mirror and ask yourself, what do I want to do everyday for the rest of my life...do that."
—Gary Vaynerchuk

When you are creating your future, you don't have time to judge you.

Chapter 3
The Birth of No Judgment Diet™

"What if you could see your naked body in the mirror and instead of tossing judgment, ridicule, and self-hatred your way, you could actually smile with gratitude at the image looking back at you?" —Katherine McIntosh

How the concept was born

There I was, standing in the hallway, bent over, grunting, skinny jeans only half way up my thighs, and it happened…again. I started panicking. My heart was pounding out of my chest, my face was flushed, and I felt heat coming off my skin like a dog in heat. I tried to control myself and hold back the tears, but without any warning the floodgates of frustration poured out of me.

I looked up at myself in the mirror and hurled a barrage of judgments at my reflection. That all-too-familiar critic had no mercy, no compassion, no sympathy. I had just had a baby two months ago! Like...give yourself a break.

But there is no break from the ridicule of the ego when it is in self-destruct mode. There I was, judging the size of my thighs, my lopsided boobs, and the fact that I couldn't fit into my skinny jeans. All of the sudden, in the middle of my body horror, I looked over at my two month old infant son on the floor beaming at me with adoration, joy, smiles, and glee. At that moment, a light bulb went off. His joy hit me instantaneously and I thought, "HOLY SHIT!"

I had spent my entire adolescent and adult life thinking my body was the root of my unhappiness. That if only I could change my body, my life would be perfect. If I just spent five plus minutes missing out on receiving my son's gratitude, joy, and adoration, I wondered what else I had spent the last 20 years of my life missing out on because I was so convinced that the person staring back at me in the mirror was ugly, fat, and ultimately unloveable. It was insane!

It was one of those moments that still to this day I remember so clearly: the sun filtering through the windows and the look of my son on our tan shag carpet. What's even more striking (and embarrassing) about that moment was I was so consumed in the downward spiral that I completely FORGOT about my son!

It was the fierce mama bear in me that didn't just want to change this 20 year destructive pattern for myself. I didn't want my son to grow up with a mom who was telling him how amazing he is while simultaneously not believing it about herself. I knew I had to make a radical shift and that there was no more time to waste. At that moment I looked at my son, and then at myself in the mirror, and I thought…

"I am going on a year-long No Judgment Diet!"

"No matter what it takes, no matter how it looks, this pattern changes NOW!" Just like my 30 day ice cream diet, I set parameters for myself. No matter what, I wasn't allowed to look in the mirror and entertain any judgment about my body. In fact, every time I did, I had to put my hand up to the mirror, look at myself, and say "STOP!" And then, immediately after, I had to find something about my body I was grateful for.

> *"Gratitude is the key to producing miracles."*
> *—Gary Douglas*

Now, this was tough for me. Finding even one thing to be grateful for about my body was a near-impossible task. So I started with the one part of my body I didn't have much judgment of: my face. I was able to have gratitude for my smile, my freckles, my skin, and my eyes. But that was about it. I could not find anything from the head down to be grateful for.

That is, until I spent a year in the mirror forcing myself to create a different story. Before that year, I never believed I could be grateful for my body. From the age of 15 I had been able to see myself only through the eyes of judgment. I saw myself as a hideous creature rather than the athletic blonde I actually was.

Once I started to finally find things I could be grateful for, it wasn't a "fake it until you make it" exercise. It was a "let me truly find something I can really be grateful for" exercise.

So there I was, skinny jeans around mid thigh, seeing through the lens of judgment, staring in the mirror...and there was a demand in my world so LOUD that I could no longer push it to the side. "NO!" I said. "STOP IT!" And there were whispers of, *there is a different way you've never tried before.*

You see, I had tried every diet, pill, tea, and exercise routine I could find; I had tried starvation, thigh master, and late night infomercials; I had tried every meditation and breathing technique under the sun. If it promised peace of mind and weight loss, I paid for it, I flew overseas for it, I considered liposuctions and surgeries for it. I spent weeks isolated in my house, afraid that if I went in public I would get judged as fat and ugly. (Newsflash: the only one judging me was me.) I was down right paranoid and obsessed with the idea that I was fat and ugly. I tortured myself, depressed myself, and did anything to AVOID looking at myself as someone who was beautiful.

That light bulb moment in the mirror with my son changed my life. For an entire year, I put myself on a No Judgment Diet. I wanted to see what else I was missing out on, what else I could create. And I simply did not want to miss out on one more minute enjoying the gift my son was because I was so selfishly focused on beating myself up in the mirror.

I spent 20 years in the pattern of ridiculing myself and my body. Nothing I did changed it permanently. All those years looking for the next thing that would change my body only made me depressed, insecure, and constantly searching for something outside of myself that I was never going to find. I had to go inside for the change.

The No Judgment Diet felt drastic, scary, and exciting. I stopped dieting and began to question the thoughts underneath every decision I've ever made about my body, food, and exercise. What happened was truly invigorating. It was a practice, and it took determination to choose.

Every time I looked at myself in the mirror and started down the rabbit hole of ridicule, I stopped. Sometimes I was already deep into it and as soon as I caught it, I stopped. I would take a moment to walk away, and I would force myself to think of a positive thought or an accomplishment about my body.

> *"Every time you have the chance to go into judgment of you or someone else, and you choose not to, you change the world."* —Dr Dain Heer

When the thought, "I hate that I can't wear a size 2" popped up, I stopped it and changed it to something positive: "I have really pretty eyes, I like my smile, I'm a strong athlete, I have an amazing son, I birthed a baby at home, these legs scored the game winning goal my senior year in highschool to get our team to win the state championship, these legs have hiked and biked mountains all over the world."

Anything that focused on and energized the gift of my body started to change and rewire the neurotransmitters. It started to initiate a new habit. I stopped waking up depressed and heavy; I began to notice I had way more energy. I stopped ridiculing my body and started to be curious about it. For the first time in 20 years, I had gratitude for my beautiful body and I started to see that it wasn't nearly as ugly and hideous as I had convinced myself it was.

I had to practice.

Just like studying a new subject, beginning a meditation practice, or starting a new exercise routine, I had to practice the habit of not judging myself. I had to practice the habit of not indulging in negative self-talk. It didn't come naturally, and it wasn't always easy. But what happened after all that practice is the reason I'm sharing my story.

If you are someone who has struggled with food, your body, or addiction, if you have secretly hated yourself or your body, I am here to say, *I've been there*. I've been there to the point that I didn't want to be here anymore. I spent 20 years and over $250,000 desperately seeking a solution to my own self-tortured ways. I didn't realize that the answer I had been looking for was inside me all along.

Following the light bulb moment with my son, something in me really began to shift. It didn't happen overnight. I didn't take a miracle pill. Instead, I practiced the art of letting go of all of the things that felt heavy. I started to realize that even though judgment about my body invaded every moment of my day, I didn't have to be a victim to the judgment. I started to have a choice with it. I could either pay attention to it or I could dismiss it and continue to move forward.

What surprised me the most about changing my relationship to judgment was not only did I get to eat the things I loved (like bacon, cheese, and ice cream) and lose weight and feel healthier, sexier, and prettier, but I actually had all of this energy to create my life. I was inspired.

When you are inspired to create, you don't have time to judge you.

We entertain judgment only when we are bored or stagnant. It's part of the reason why many successful people consistently wear the same outfit over and over again: they want to eliminate any need to overthink or judge their wardrobe. Creation and forward momentum is the priority, not judgment or dwelling on the past.

Once I started to see that judgment was a choice, it no longer weighed on me like a ton of bricks. If you've ever been around judgment, you know how heavy it can be. Judgment is one of the main culprits of weight gain and can also be the reason many people struggle with losing weight. Have you ever tried going on a diet and you barely ate anything but your body still gained weight? I sure did. I see clients all the time who are so confused because they eat barely anything and still gain weight.

Why?

Because judgments weigh a ton. When you are eating salad and judging you as inadequate, overweight, or not enough, your body will gain weight—not from the food but from the judgments. To be clear, I'm not saying that you should eat whatever you want and not pay attention to what you actually require. This is about connecting with what's true for you. Paying attention to the big and small cues your body gives you... but doing it with awareness, not judgment. There is a big difference: judgments solidify and create density while awareness creates lightness.

I was shocked when eating ice cream for 30 days resulted in me losing 10 pounds. The reason I lost the weight is because after the fourth or fifth day I started to remove the judgments I had about ice cream. I started to ENJOY every single bite without any judgment. When that happened, I actually ate less ice cream. Every bite was like a happy dance. I was so thoroughly in the moment, it was ecstasy every day. That is what created the change.

If you have spent your whole life looking for the thing that's going to help you and you have felt hopeless or like giving up, I am here to share with you a different way. **It's not an answer so much as it is an invitation to discover the strength, power, and beauty inside of you that you have been hiding from you and the world.**

When you commit to letting go of judging you, your body, and your food choices, you can begin to open up a whole new world. What changed my life was, instead of just surviving, I started to create a future that I had always dreamed of...but had no idea how to get there.

> *"The future belongs to those who believe in the beauty of their dreams." —Eleanor Roosevelt*

I always wanted to have a business where I got to contribute to people's physical and mental health, but I never thought I could create a six-figure business doing that. Yet just 10 short months after starting my year-long No Judgment Diet, I had created a six-figure income doing what I LOVED. I was having so much fun creating, and, in the process, I saved my mortgage, saved my family from filing for bankruptcy, created a global business, and traveled the world with my husband and son (who, at the end of those 10 months, had just turned 1).

I had accomplished two things I had deemed IMPOSSIBLE: I completely changed my relationship with my body <u>and</u> I created a profitable business that allowed me to travel the world, bring my son with me, and do what I love. It was a dream come true.

Since the age of 15 I knew I wanted to do something with bodies. I wanted to work on them and activate the body's own healing capacities. Yet even though that's what I always knew I wanted to do, I never thought I could make a good living doing it. So I always chose professions that would produce enough income that I could do energy work on the side. The problem was, I never had enough energy left after working 60-80-100 hours a week.

The experience of creating my own job and my own career showed me that I could do what I love <u>and</u> get paid more than I thought possible.

It taught me there is a different way.

Prior to embarking on my year-long No Judgment Diet, I never thought I would get free of the mental hell I had put myself through. I simply didn't know that I could change it. I didn't know that the answer *wasn't* in a diet, a pill, an exercise routine, a book, a master's degree in psychology, the therapist's office, a mood disorder pill, or anything else. The answer to setting me free from my own constraints came from unlocking the wrongness and misconceptions of my own hidden insecurities.

Gary Douglas, one of my mentors and the founder of Access Consciousness®, says, "You're not as screwed up as you think." Similarly, Dr. Dain Heer, the co-founder, has said that after almost 20 years of facilitating this material all over the world, there is not one person he has come across that is actually more screwed up than they think. Every single one of them has seen that they are brighter, more talented, more beautiful, smarter, and more aware than they have ever given themselves credit for.

There *is* a possibility for a different solution.

One that begins to address the joy and beauty of you—instead of the focus being on changing your physical body. And the crazy thing is, when you begin to let go of the judgments and the rigid conclusions of what your body can and can't eat, should and shouldn't eat, and how much time it needs to exercise, the molecules of your body begin to change. You will begin to have more freedom in how you see yourself and the world around you. This isn't a quick fix; this is a way to get you to start enjoying the journey of living.

An elephant doesn't hide behind a tree because it doesn't want people to admire its behind. A giraffe doesn't cut off its neck. A hippo doesn't think it's too big. A dog doesn't complain about having too many spots.

Us humans come in all shapes and sizes. To think there are body types, sizes, shapes, and colors that are better than the rest prevents us from celebrating our differences. We are all made up of different genetic, mental, and physical material. Why would our bodies be any different?

Isn't it time you started to embrace the skin you're in, to be the beauty you truly be?

If not now, when?

Chapter 4
The Beginning of Something Different

"It's not about getting to a number on a scale - it's about creating a vision for how you want your life to look."
—Oprah

Could you imagine what your life would be like if you never had to diet or worry about a number on a scale again?

If you can't, you are not alone. In fact, you are among the hundreds of millions of people searching for the answer that will give them the body they think they want. But the reality is, most people don't want to diet or measure their happiness based on a number. Deep down most people just want to be happy. They want peace of mind. They want to feel fulfilled. They want meaningful experiences. They want to be enough and they truly desire to be the best version of themselves they can be.

Most people go on a diet because they think that losing weight will make them happy. They think that losing weight will make them feel better and give them the confidence they think they lack. But here's the deal: if you think you need to lose weight then you have to judge all the things you think are wrong with you. And then you have to judge whether or not you're getting it right.

That's a whole lot of judgment. And what's even worse, when you are judging you, then you begin to see things through the eyes of judgment. That is no way to live. As long as you are judging you, you cannot be aware of what you know, you cannot open the door to a new experience, and you cannot receive anything that doesn't match your judgments.

Years ago, I was bartending & waiting tables while dating the man who would eventually become my husband and the father of my son. We had been together for a couple years and we also happened to work together. I was having an off day, feeling sorry for myself. Per usual, I felt fat, ugly, and unattractive. I was judging myself hardcore and I literally could not hear anyone or anything that was said that didn't match my poor pathetic judgment of myself that I was fat, ugly, and unattractive.

There was a moment, where he came over to me and said, did you hear that?

I replied: "Hear What?"

He said: "That person just complimented you".

My response: "No they didn't".

What ensued was a back and forth banter between the two of us in which he was trying to convince me that I receive more compliments than anyone he had ever met in his life. The only problem is: I could never hear them because they didn't match my judgments I had of myself.

As a young adult, I remember being at family gatherings and social settings and people would always compliment me, and I just remember thinking in my head that they were just doing that to be nice. They were lying to me and they didn't really mean it. I literally could not hear anything that didn't match my judgments of myself.

Judgment is not a creative energy. It keeps limitations in place. It is heavy and it usually perpetuates depression, anxiety, low self-esteem, poor decision making and so much more. Is it fun for you to hang out with people who are judging you all the time? No, because it is hard to feel inspired under such duress.

But imagine for a moment, spending your time with people who don't judge you, they believe in you, they believe in who you are and what you do...

Would you have more energy to create your life?

Choosing to eliminate judgment from your life allows you to have choice; it opens the door to possibilities. This is where living begins to take place. When you decide you aren't going to "diet" but instead choose a more conscious path of creating with your body, your entire world can change. When we are invested in judgment it is hard to change, it is hard to be inspiring, it is hard to go outside of ourselves, and it is hard to access that creative energy that never stops. Judgment breeds a place where there is little choice and little room for growth.

> *"As long as you are doing judgment instead of choice, nothing will ever change."*
> *—Gary Douglas*

That's a huge statement. It means that if you are judging yourself in order to change your body, you will never truly have the change you desire. And what's more, you won't be able to be aware of the different choices you can choose because those choices don't match your judgments. As long as you hold on to judgments and points of view that keep limitations in place, lasting change can't happen.

Does the body have a point of view? No. But you have a point of view about your body. Every point of view you have about your body, your body will prove your point of view right.

For example: If you decide your body is fat, your body will create a fat body to prove your point of view is correct. If you decide you can't, your body will prove you are correct. If you decide you have a slow metabolism, your body will create a slow metabolism. What you think and feel is what you create.

There is another way.

I am here to invite you to let go of the idea that you need to lose weight, and instead to embrace the idea that if you start loving your body and begin to have total gratitude for it, you can transform both your body and your life.

When you stop obsessing about change via judgment, you can begin to obsess about the things that you are wildly passionate about. When you focus on what you're passionate about, what drives you, what gets you out of bed in the mornings, then you have energy to create your life. Food, your body image, and your obsession about your body becomes far less critical in distracting you from what really matters.

And that is where the magic is. Things grow where your attention goes. So if you are constantly thinking about all the things you think are wrong with you, you get more things wrong with you.

If you start to shift your attention and begin to see and receive your body through the eyes of gratitude, complete change is possible. Gratitude is one of the highest vibrations on the planet. Einstein said you cannot solve a problem in the same way you created it. It makes sense that you will not be able to solve the problem you think you have with your body by perpetrating judgment.

When you make the choice to go on a diet, is it because you have gratitude for your body? Or are you making that choice from a state of judging you and judging that something needs to change? True change does not occur by focusing on the problem. True change occurs by focusing on the possibilities, by shifting your perspective, and by choosing something different.

Every time you choose something different, or you shift a habit, you rewire your neurotransmitters. And when you rewire your brain, you begin to see things you've never seen before. However, if you continue to bang your head against the same door, the door to a different possibility remains closed no matter how many times you open it.

In my first year of grad school, I was like an optimistic little kid: bright eyed, full of enthusiasm, and eager to learn. I couldn't wait! The information felt fresh and exciting. I devoured the information. I studied, experimented, and took initiative to research anything that had to do with the body, psychology, and the possibilities for transformation. I volunteered to become my own subject for the purpose of experimenting. Every waking hour was consumed by any topic that opened the door to show the connection between the body and mind.

Candace Pert is known for uncovering the fact that there are more brain cells in your gut. Hence why there is actual truth to the saying: trust your gut. After the initial excitement wore off, the reality of needing to follow the guidelines within the school structure set in.

As a part of the curriculum, we were required to personally attend therapy. And that's where the downward spiral started to unravel within me. I forced myself to look for and talk about and explore the problems about my body and in a very short amount of time, I started to lose myself. I started to binge eat, obsess about my body, make myself wrong, and I found myself so deep into my old destructive habits that I felt like I was drowning.

My excitement to consume new content got replaced by my all too familiar obsession to hate my body, binge eat, self-sabotage, hide, and obsessively envelop myself in a blanket of shame so thick that I almost suffocated myself to death. Every day, we were forced to "look at" our problems. We had to talk about our problems, listen to our fellow peers' problems. We had to journal about it, write papers on it, meditate on it, move with it, and talk to our teachers and therapists about it.

It was no wonder that by the end of my first year of grad school I had officially hit rock bottom. I was binge eating at least two pints of Ben & Jerry's Ice Cream in secret more frequently than I care to admit. 10 pounds later, I was an emotional train wreck, and desperate to climb myself out of my own self-induced hell hole. I diagnosed myself as the most depressed I had ever been in my entire life.

I wanted to die. Focusing on the things you think you need to change, will never truly invite and inspire true change. But focusing on something that inspires you, gets you out of bed in the morning, leaves you thinking about it non stop because every time you do, it energizes you, now that is the kind of change that dreams are made of.

What would this life be like if you enjoyed your body?

Imagine choosing a diet from a place of total gratitude for your body? If you are choosing that, then by all means, go on as many diets as you desire! However, if you are choosing a diet to restrict, judge, and cut out joy, then maybe it's time for a different kind of diet. One where you eliminate judgment, and add in possibilities. One of my favorite questions to ask when transforming the body is to ask: What can I add into my daily life?

More water? More vegetables? More movement? More adventures? Doesn't that sound like a better diet to go on? Joy is possible when you truly begin to understand the way your body works. You are an amazing being. Your body is a vibrant, living, breathing gift. And you are only given one body in this lifetime.

Most of us learned to think that our body is a problem that needs to be controlled. We aren't taught how to honor it and treat it well. We aren't taught to believe that our body is a gift. We are taught to judge it, push it, stuff it, order it around, and drag it through our lives. We are taught that food makes our bodies fat or fit. But food does not create our bodies as much as you would like to believe. Judgments create our bodies.

Ouch. That doesn't sound like very much fun, does it?

What if you chose to explore a different relationship with you and your body?

This may seem like a far out concept, but these ideas come from over 20 years teaching movement classes, extensive studies in Somatic Psychology, personal experience, a voracious appetite for all things unseen, traveling all over the world and seeing how much the world judges themselves, and the deep desire to offer a way of living and being that actually works long term and empowers people to trust that they know.

I studied teachers and teachings from all walks of life. The things that created the most change, the quickest, never delivered an answer, but offered a possibility. When you discover what works for you, then no one can take it away from you. A question will always empower you to know what you know. A conclusion is a judgment and usually requires you to align and agree or resist and react to it. But when you discover what is true for you on your own, it has a lightness to it that no one can take away from you.

I never thought in a million years that I could have peace of mind with my body. From once being anorexic, bulimic, and deeply troubled with my body, to now truly loving the skin I'm in. It has changed my whole life.

I have so much more confidence in myself. I trust that I can create and have and do and be anything I want. I know what foods actually work for me and which ones slow me down or temporarily stifle my confidence. But the most significant change is that I trust myself. I no longer go searching outside of myself for the answer. I always know that the truth I am seeking for myself is just one question away.

I have taught myself the different ways in which my body communicates with me and all the different ways in which my body seeks to heal itself. Through goosebumps, gut instincts, cool breezes, heart palpitations, random bouts of temporary pain (lasting just a few short seconds at this point), yawns, random noises, eye twitches, throat changes, sensory experiences.

This journey helped me change the things I cannot change. And if you stick with it, and become your own private investigator, devouring content that helps you reveal your own truth, you too will change the things you thought you couldn't and you will drastically change your body and the way you live in it in the world.

The target is to create a different world with the way we live in our bodies.

I tried so many things before. I studied for a master's degree in Somatic Psychology, went to therapy, was in and out of eating disorder clinics, tried every diet I could think of, studied Shamanism, and did over 100 soul retrievals and past life regressions. I tried dancing it out and talking it out. I tried doing reiki, hypnotism, massage, energy work, body talk, mud baths, cleanses, and colonics. Although some of the above did help me create a deeper sense of self, at the end of the day I still felt like something was missing. I still felt like my body was wrong.

I didn't think it was possible to truly LOVE my body, to no longer see it as a problem, to no longer judge it as a wrongness. I thought it was impossible...that no way in a million years could I change this.

And yet, one day, after many days, weeks, and months practicing the concepts in The No Judgment Diet, the deep-seeded wrongness disappeared and I started to truly LOVE my body. Is it perfect? NO. Do I let myself have chocolate and bacon? YES (as much as possible). Do I love sugar and ice cream? YES. And I also love greens, vegetables, tea, and lemon water. I love to move my body as much as possible. I love to exercise and play outdoors. But more importantly I realize there is so much more to living than spending my life judging my body, food, and a few extra pounds.

The No Judgment Diet creates the possibility for you to truly love your body and to find true happiness in your life. It won't tell you what to do, but instead it invites you to discover what's true for you. When you know what's true for you, no one can take your truth away from you.

This is about freedom. Freedom to love your body. Freedom to choose. Freedom to no longer make judgment relevant. Freedom to make a different choice. This isn't about what is right or wrong. This isn't about whether to diet or not to diet. This is about what you can choose and do that lights you up and simultaneously nurtures you and your body. When you are nurturing your body, you are living your life and you have space to create your life.

Your body is not a judgeable offense. Every time you judge your body, you cut off the contribution you can be in the world. You'll never hear an elephant complain about the size of its ass or see it hide behind a bush because it doesn't want to be seen. Elephants are a gift just by being. Imagine if they had judgments. If they did, we wouldn't be able to receive the gift they are.

Every judgment you have of your body prevents you from receiving the gift it came into the world to be. Now is your time to choose something different. To truly let go of all the old patterning and programming. Stop looking for reasons to judge you and start looking for ways you could create. When we look for things that are wrong, we find things that are wrong. When we look for things that are right, we find things that are right.

When it comes to your body, how can you apply this principle to benefit you?

Your body desires to contribute to you. It desires to have your back. It desires to have fun, be light and carefree and truly enjoy living!

It is not purposefully out to get you, or make you gain weight, or create discomfort within you. However when those things happen, it is simply the body's way of trying to facilitate you to shift your perspective, change your point of view, and take a different course of action.

Can you imagine what it would be like to receive the idea that your body has your back? What would it be like if you had your body's back? Get curious and stop judging you. You *got* this!

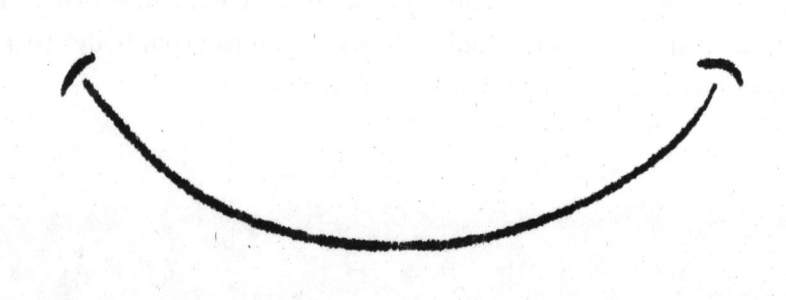

Chapter 5
Go On a Date... with Your Body!

"The hardest part about change is making a new choice."
—Joe Dispenza

Can you imagine what your life would be like if you treated your body with the same curiosity and admiration as someone you are interested in?

Do you know what your body wants? Does your body know what you want? If you were in a long term relationship with your body, would it last?

I know this might sound like a foreign concept, but the truth is, your body is the longest lasting relationship you will ever have. It is with you through thick and thin, but the challenge with this relationship is it is usually one sided.

Your body is usually at the effect of your wants, needs, and demands. But think about what would happen if you began to include your body. Imagine what your life would be like if you truly leaned into creating a greater future with your body?

The key to relationships is communication, listening, negotiating, appreciating, compromising, and gratitude! It's about surrendering enough into allowing your body to communicate…

Your body is always communicating in sensations, feelings, goosebumps, chills, sweats, pains, and so much more!

Are you willing to listen?

When you feel pain, or there's a pit in your stomach, or you get goosebumps, or it feels like a cool breeze moves through your body, or someone shakes your hand and you get a feeling…those are just a few examples from the hundreds of different ways your body is speaking to you.

We've all had times when we chose something against our better judgment only to discover later that our gut instinct was right. Most people, in that moment, deep inside themselves, say, "I knew it!"

The challenge with listening to the body is that it requires a deep internal trust of oneself. It's not that the body talks back in words, but it is always communicating. Like a relationship, the more time you spend with someone, the more you get to understand the unspoken energies. The more you listen to your body and you understand the energies, you can create a lasting relationship with your body and little by little you will lean into the way you & your body are most effective together.

Your body's primary language is energy.

Bodies do not speak the language of words. If your body could speak in words it would probably be screaming at you and saying something that may be hard to hear. **The body's language, the language of energy, is subtle, like a whisper, and when you tune in and take a moment to listen you will discover a whole new way of living...**where you and your body become an unstoppable duo of possibility, change, transformation, lightness, and joy.

In contrast, when you ignore your body's subtle cues, it starts to turn up the volume. And when you keep ignoring it, it turns up the volume even more. It gets louder and louder and louder, like a little kid trying to get his mom's attention, until you can no longer ignore your body's way of trying to get your attention. It may show up as pain, weight gain, disease, loss of hearing or sight, skin disorders, immune deficiencies, hair loss, depression, stress, anxiety, and so much more.

Why do most of us spend so much time ignoring our bodies? Because we don't want to hear the sad, hard truth, that for the majority of our lives, we have been ignoring our bodies. We haven't learned to be curious about our bodies' likes and dislikes. We haven't been taught to listen, be curious, have gratitude, and invite our bodies to be one of our greatest co-creators in life.

It's not your fault. We're not taught to listen to it. We're taught to be a dictator—directing it, bossing it, beating it, and judging it. Your body has been around the block with you for a number of decades, so you start taking it for granted. You ignore it. You get tired of it. You drag it around. You wake up and judge it. Imagine the most intimate relationship you have in your life was like this…

You wake up and the person that supposedly cares the most for you, has nothing but gratitude for you, and wants to see you succeed starts nagging at you, judging you, and telling you that you are not enough. It makes a huge impact and creates significant distance between you and the person you are with.

Your body is no different. **It is the longest and most permanent relationship you'll have in this lifetime.** It is always there for you—thick or thin, rain or shine, depressed or happy. No matter your mood it has never left your side.

What would your life be like if you started to wake up every day and realize that your body is your most loyal companion? What if you thanked it for weathering all the storms with you? What if you stopped taking it for granted and, like a first date, got curious about its needs, wishes, and desires?

Think about a first date. You are curious, excited, and nervous. You look your best. You pay attention. You are present to everything. You might start future tripping, or inventing stories, but you always try to come back to the moment.

Imagine if you treated a first date as something to be taken for granted? You dressed sloppy, slouched, had bad manners, and weren't polite. Your chances of a second date are slim to none.

Let me give you an example.

A couple years ago, I was enjoying being single and was dating a lot. The dating scene in the age of dating apps and swiping left or right was new to me. It was fascinating; I called it "shopping for my reality." I wanted to see what was out there. Being someone who was now an independent, single mom, who had been married twice and divorced twice, I identified some relationship patterns I wanted to change.

I knew I had to look within, not outside, to change those patterns. I was the common denominator. I had recognized that my genius was to masterfully become whomever someone needed me to be. (Side note from my psychology studies: My relationship pattern of becoming whatever someone needed me to be was based on survival mechanisms I learned as an empathic kid.) I was still being me, but I would adapt my needs, wishes, and desires to match their life. I showed up so fully for their dreams, that our hearts would connect and the miracle of intimacy would transform both of us. But part of me was always missing.

The challenge in almost every relationship we have is to maintain a sense of self, encourage self growth and expansion and aliveness while growing, expanding, and developing the relationship. Unfortunately, many people either start cutting off parts of themselves to get in a relationship or to stay in the relationship.

Eventually I started to give credence to my own wishes and desires. As I showed up fully for my dreams and allowed those dreams to be part of the relationship, the relationship would change. Without fail, my newfound passion for my dreams surprised both of my husbands and disrupted the long-term stability of our connection, creating separation, frustration, and confusion that ultimately led to the demise of each relationship. As I began to date again, I knew I wanted a relationship that could fully accommodate my dreams as well as support and grow with me through all of my changes.

But how?

I knew I had to start a relationship with my dreams included from the start. Part of what went wrong was that I failed to share what I wanted and needed from the beginning. This is HUGE! I expected it to be okay to show up for them, do all the right things, make them think that I was happy as is. But that wasn't true. So when I started to voice my dreams, there was conflict and that was all on me. Moving forward I knew I needed to start including my dreams from the beginning.

I learned that most people fall in love with the personality or characteristics of a person. But life is always changing and we are always transforming and tweaking our likes and dislikes, our personality.

But our core values, the truth of who we actually are, tends to remain consistent. So the invitation is to fall in love with who the person is, not what they do. That is where lasting long term fulfilling relationships develop... fall in love with the being, not their characteristics.

The same is true for your body. Your body is going to feel different at 55 than it did at 25. Fall in love with the values and the core of your body, and your body will support you. Judge your body through its changes because it's characteristics change over time and it will be more challenging for you to change with your body and for your body to change with you.

Creating The Future

> *"The biggest adventure you can ever take*
> *is to live the life of your dreams."*
> —Oprah Winfrey

As a single woman in my early 40s, I knew who I was. I knew what I wanted my future to look like. I knew how important my dreams were to me, and I knew I was willing to do absolutely anything and everything to make those dreams come true. Through my own experience I knew the life-transforming phenomenon of letting go of judgment of the body, and I knew it was a revolutionary experience that could truly change the planet.

If I could go from judging, obsessing, resisting, reacting, and restricting to a life of being alive, awake, successful, motivated, traveling the world with my family, and feeling a sense of freedom, I knew that it was possible for women all over the planet. The more I did what I loved, the more fun and money appeared everywhere I went…I knew this could literally change the world.

Remember that only 4 percent of women worldwide consider themselves beautiful?

That means 96 percent of the women on the planet are living a life of judgment and are suppressing the possibility of freedom in every area of their life. That means their productivity at work suffers, their relationships suffer, their sex lives suffer, their children suffer, and so much more.

(Living a life of judgment also applies to men, of course, but men are less likely to talk about the issues they have with their bodies so there aren't many statistics out there. My experience has been that almost every man I've known was either thinking about or talking about changing their body in some way.)

The truth is both men and women make excuses or justify their perceived body's fallacies. But what if, as a world, we looked for the brilliance of the body, the capacities of the body. What if we didn't first look for the flaws? What if instead, we celebrated the greatness? Would that change the world?

Imagine if every person on the planet loved their body?

> *"Imperfection is beauty, madness is genius and it's better to be absolutely ridiculous than absolutely boring."*
> —*Marilyn Monroe*

Imagine if no one worried about the size of their thighs. Imagine if no one used food to numb their pain. Obesity is a disease where people cut off their awareness and stay addicted to the judgments they have about themselves.

Intimacy suffers when people judge their bodies. In my experience, women have sex with men when they feel good about themselves. And a large percentage of the female population does not feel good about themselves based on how they perceive and feel in their bodies. So they withdraw from sex and intimacy, which leads to men feeling less masculine and less empowered. This leads to cheating, divorce, broken families, and a whole lot of unnecessary pain and suffering—all because the woman doesn't fit into her own unrealistic societal expectations of what a sexy woman looks like.

What if instead of asking to lose weight, you started asking to be the size of sexy for your body? That's a different place to live from. Insecurity is a self-imposed infliction based on women deciding they will never fit the ideal. But the "ideal' is unrealistic for probably 95 percent of the population, and even supermodels judge their bodies.

Life isn't about fitting some arbitrary aesthetic ideal; it's about being **happy, awake, and in tune** with what's true for you. I believe that **a sexy woman is one who is in love with herself.** A sexy woman has confidence, loves her body, eats cake, plays outside, and listens to and communicates her needs. True sexiness and self-confidence has nothing to do with size.

> *"Nothing makes a woman more beautiful*
> *than the belief that she is beautiful."*
> *—Sophia Loren*

You know what isn't sexy? Someone who judges their body, obsesses over food, and restricts themselves. Someone who won't receive compliments and is constantly criticizing herself and her appearance—criticism that eventually turns outward and hurts her relationships.

Think about it; how many people do you know who *don't* judge their body? How many people do you know who don't have points of views about food, sugar, diet, nutrition, or exercise? I personally don't know very many (if any) people who don't have *many* points of views about bodies and diet.

Everyone has an opinion.

It seems like most people are either on one extreme or the other: The uber-obsessive health conscious people who judge anyone who isn't a fitness freak OR the ones who want to be healthy, get fit, lose weight, but never feel like they can. However, we all know there is something in the middle.

I've been on both extremes: I spent much of my younger years obsessing over fitness and then, later in life, strongly resisting it. After I turned 15, I was obsessed with fitness yet could never find the balance between food, emotions, and my body image. It always felt off. Years later, I definitely found myself in the grocery store secretly purchasing pints of Ben & Jerry's Chubby Hubby and Cherry Garcia. That lifestyle also felt off because underneath the sneaky, hidden actions was a universe of unidentified shame.

What truly began to change my reality was my willingness to let go of any preconceived thoughts, judgments, and conclusions about what I thought I wanted my body to look like instead of what it desired to look like. Instead of following mainstream advice, I had to start paying attention to my own awareness. I had to ditch conventional wisdom and embrace non linear, non cognitive wisdom. True change comes from within.

I knew this because 20 years of doing it the logical way always made me gain weight, binge eat, obsess about food and my body, which ultimately led to a depressing roller coaster that wasn't very stable nor very fun. But when I ditched the judgments and did it my way, I lost 10 pounds in 30 days eating ice cream. That was one of my many wake up calls.

I went on a journey where I listened, got curious, and played with my way, not someone else's way. I asked questions: What food did it really want? What movements did it really crave? What clothes made my body come alive? Curiosity was a huge key to discovering what was truly possible that I had never before considered.

Prior to getting curious, I would simply decide what I thought my body NEEDED to fit my projected desired outcome. Imagine being in a relationship where your partner tells you what to eat, how to work out, what to wear, and what not to do. That would be horrible, yet that was the relationship I had with my body. I had time constraints, food constraints, diet regimens, exercise requirements, and a whole lot more that ultimately led to my breakdown. And every breakdown eventually leads to a breakthrough. Once I got curious and realized this concept, I started to ASK A LOT OF QUESTIONS.

Instead of asking, "Body, what do you want to eat?"—which is vague and boring, kind of like asking a date, "What do you like?"—I started asking different questions, ones that engaged curiosity and were more specific.

Please feel free to write the questions below down and carry them in your phone or put them in your kitchen, or hang them on your bathroom mirror. The more you get comfortable with asking, the more you can recognize your own ability to be a good listener. Pay attention to the energy you get back, and then follow your knowing.

The body will commuicate in all types of ways. The invitation isn't to get it right every time, but rather perceive, feel, and listen to the energetic cues. Kind of like when you meet someone and there is an energy between you, this applies to lovers, friends, business connections, someone who helps you at a store and so much more. Pay attention to the subtle cues and you will have a better understanding of all the different ways your body is communicating to you. The majority of communication (70 - 93%) is non verbal. When applied to the body, it is almost always communicating non verbally, but you can pay attention to subtle cues like, does your heart open, do you cross your arms, do you lean forward, or lean back, do you get goosebumps or butterflies in your stomach or do you feel like you just got punched in the gut? You can also pay attention to your sounds, throat and mouth. Whenever I am facilitating, I notice the partcipants body language and I especially pay attention to what I'm saying and how the particpants are reacting. Are they smiling? Do they laugh when I say something that is true for them? Are they leaning back, shaking their head, have a stern look, did they gasp, are they nodding their head? These are all the ways the body communicates, so practice listening, sensing, feeling as you ask qurstions and you will discover a whole new world of possibilities that can translate accross your entire life.

Remember, this is a lifelong process of forming a new relationship with yourself and your body where you get to empower yourself, listen, and get acquainted with a whole new way of relating. Here is an example of some of the questions you can ask. Please feel free to make a list of your own! And then remember to practice paying attention to how you and your body respond to these questions. It isn't about getting it right or perfect, it's about putting it into practice. So have fun practicing. You got this!

Body, what foods would make you feel sexy?

Body, what foods would give you the energy of abundance?

Body, what foods would turn you on?

Body, what foods would make you more money?

Body, what foods would give you more energy?

Body, what foods would energize you today?

Those questions were much more interesting. Asking them started to create an energetic dialogue that not only changed my body but began attracting energies, people, and money into my life that matched where I wanted to go and what I wanted to create in the world.

What I had never realized until I got curious was all of my opinions and projections about food I had been told since I was little *were all judgments*. And judgments destroy possibilities.

Every judgment you do of you takes you out of being the source for life and living. It also takes you out of being present and distracts you from creating the future you truly desire to have.

Your body will create itself if you are willing to create with it, connect with it, be curious, ask it questions, have gratitude for it, and stop concluding that you know better. No one likes a know-it-all. No one likes to be around someone who thinks they know better. So just like your most intimate relationship, what would happen if you started to treat your body like you would your favorite person in the whole wide world?

Relationships, and healthy thriving relationships are a great window into how to create a different reality with your body. Think about it… what kinds of relationships would you like to have with yourself, your friends, your intimate others, your partners, your spouses? What would feel most nurturing and alive for you?

When I was newly single I really had to get curious and discover what would really work for me? I had two failed marriages, and a live-in relationship that ended in disaster. It would be easy to blame it on "them". But the truth was: I was the common denominator in every single one of those experiences. This concept applies to the body. Your thoughts are the common denominator in every diet plan or exercise plan you've ever chosen. Perhaps, like my failed relationships, it wasn't their fault, just like it's not the diet's fault.

What was I bringing to the table that was creating conflict, pain, and sabotage? What was inside of me that was creating so much turmoil? I went on a very intense self-reflective journey to heal the hidden pain, to uncover the reasons I was the way I was, and to find much more healthy ways of navigating my own shortcomings.

I also wanted to discover what I actually desired. Was I willing to give myself permission to truly have it all? Even if I had no clue where to start or how to discover what I desired, the entrepreneur, the rebel, the future-thinker in me wondered: "If I don't see any examples of what I truly desire, what if I gave myself permission to discover what was true for me and then just created it?"

So I went on a series of dates to explore what I actually wanted. I went shopping for my reality. And I stayed curious.

And at the end of seven first dates, most of the men, at one point during the course of the date, said in a joking tone, "Will you marry me?" or "Where have you been all my life?" or "I think you're my dream girl." Yet I walked away from each and every one of those dates thinking, "I'm not even sure I want a *second* date." I didn't have a second date with any of them.

It was a real wake-up call for me.

What the heck was I doing to make these men be totally infatuated with me?

I realized that exact pattern was how I landed two husbands: I was brilliant at fitting myself into other people's realities. The problem was, eventually I was left feeling empty, confused, hurt, and dissatisfied because without realizing it I had left my reality behind. It was all about them. I was completely willing to show up for them and do whatever it took to keep them happy; I would support their dreams, show up for their careers, and sacrifice my plans in favor of theirs. I would stay up late, wake up early, and do whatever it took for whatever they needed. I would cook and clean and work and make sacrifices. I would laugh and joke and say "Yes" to them and "No" to friends or any personal obligations I had. I put their happiness and their needs in front of mine. Then, at last, this giant, vacant hole in my heart led me to the profound realization that I was never willing to look at what *I* wanted or needed.

I had never given myself permission to have needs or even entertain them. My sole purpose was to sacrifice myself for someone else's happiness. This "aha" moment was a huge turning point in my life.

I finally realized and acknowledged that I had sacrificed myself for the peace and happiness of others. I would be whatever they needed me to be whenever they needed me to be it. I fit myself into their world. I was adaptable, and I was brilliant at it. But when it came time to develop my own interests, most of the relationships would fade away.

When it came time to ask for what I wanted, I honestly didn't know. When it was time to be me, I didn't know how. I was so consumed in being what they wanted me to be that I abandoned myself in favor of their needs. And the especially sad part was, I had no idea I was doing it!

So, having finally realized this, I started to take *myself* on dates. I would bring a notebook and ask myself questions I had never considered asking before:

What did *I* want?

What were *my* dreams?

What was important to *me*?

What could *I* live with?

What were *my* non-negotiables and *my* deal breakers?

Where was *I* willing to compromise?

What were the areas that were really important to *me*?

Would I be willing to ask for what I want?

This exercise in taking myself on dates was another wake-up call. Had I really spent the majority of my adult life trying to make others happy without any consideration for what would make *me* happy? I really thought that my happiness and purpose in life was predicated on whether or not *they* were happy.

Asking for what *you* want is one of the core principles in beginning to create the life you desire. So please feel free to take the above list and take yourself on a date. Add to the list, discover what is important to you, not just in your intimate relationships, but what is actually important to you with yourself and your body. What are your non-negotiables? What are your body's non-negotiables? This is a relationship, a chance to create with your body. It is not meant to be a dictatorship.

Being in relationship with your body is a two way street. You still need to pay attention to it, be respectful and aware of all the ways it's trying to communicate with you. Ask it questions. And be in a place where you aren't judging your body so you can actually receive the information and then go execute.

But know, you can negotiate with it. Just like a long lasting intimate relationship, there is compromise, negotiation, listening, and understanding. It comes down to allowance, acceptance and gratitude. Stop judging and start listening.

What would it be like if you invested more energy in your dreams and less energy in your judgments?

Ask and you shall receive is a law of the universe. When it comes to the human body, ask for the body you want. But also be willing to ask the body what it wants to be in the world that you're not letting it be. I know it may sound foreign, but you have dreams and your body can help you make those dreams come true. Just ask, does your body know how to help you make those dreams come true? This is where the practice of listening comes into play. What do you perceive? Did your heart race? Did your palms get sweaty? Did you feel a pit in your stomach? These are all ways your body can communicate with you. So start paying attention because it will lead to greatness in every area of your life! This is where ideas come to fruition!

Most of us were not taught to receive information from our bodies. We were taught to work hard, exercise it, sleep it, feed it, ignore it, put a bandaid on it, stuff it, shut it, even starve it. We were taught if it's in pain, to go to the doctor, listen to an outside authority, follow instructions of that outside authority, and then give it a pill or feed it medicine. But we weren't taught to take a look at the bigger picture and see that if the body is in pain, perhaps it is trying to communicate something.

The truth is the body is always communicating to us. However most of us have been entrained to listen when the body acts out in an unpleasant way: weight gain, sickness, fatigue, pain, disease, and so much more. The reality is the body is always communicating in whispers, in subtle requests, but if we ignore it for too long, then the only way to get your attention is to turn up the volume.

Just like a little kid who is trying to get their mother's or father's attention. After being ignored a few times, the child starts to increase the volume until the parent pays attention. The body does the same thing.

If you really want a different body, first change the way you relate to it. You can always go on a diet, but it is short term. True change that lasts includes living in a body you love. So, it's time to stop being so bossy, judgmental, demanding, and ungrateful towards your body and expecting it to change in a positive way.

One way to build a relationship with your body in which you could actually be happy is to take it on a first date…just like you've never met before. Imagine being able to relate to your body with fresh eyes, without a frame of reference of the past: with excitement, curiosity, and patience.

On a first date, you might be nervous, but you are also present, attentive, curious, excited, and giving it your best. Imagine being *that* present and curious with your body every day.

Many of us have had the experience of going on a date and feeling ignored. Heck, there were plenty of dates where I, out of sheer nerves and insecurity, talked too much and didn't ask enough questions.

When you go on a first date, you want the person you're on a date with to be interested in you, ask you questions, and lean in. Your date also wants you to ask them questions and be interested in them. If either of you are too demanding, judgmental, or critical of the other, there probably won't be a second date.

Can you imagine going on a first date and the person you're on the date with doesn't ask what you would like to eat or drink and just orders for you? They decide what you should have. They just start shouting orders at you. And then, in the middle of shouting orders at you, they tell you you're not good enough. You're too fat. You aren't skinny enough, fit enough, tall enough, sexy enough. You're too quiet, you're too loud, your clothes are too bright, you're dressed too conservatively. If that was your experience on the date, chances are you probably wouldn't stay there and continue to engage with this person, let alone choose to go on a second date.

Why? Because your date didn't ask you any questions. Your date ordered for you, demanded what your body was going to eat, and then judged the crap out of you and started to pick you apart. Your date did not include you or consider you at all.

Think about how we do this to our bodies everyday. We tell our bodies what they need to eat. Then we force them to eat or force them to not eat, and no matter what size or shape our bodies are, we judge them. We judge them for being too big, too small, too skinny, too tall, too short, too thick, too thin, too white, too dark, too young, too old…

Can you imagine?

Would you treat somebody you were going on a first date with the way you treat your body?

Every day, we wake up and judge our bodies, and yet every day our bodies still wake up and are here to contribute to us. However, over time, if the body isn't invited to participate in the relationship with you, it begins to fight back and break down.

Your Most Important Relationship

Nobody can tell you how to do your body.

Would your body still choose to be with you if it had the choice? If you treat your body like I used to treat mine - Probably not. No one likes to be discarded, judged, ridiculed, reprimanded, ignored, looked down upon, criticized, and treated like a slave. Your body is the same way. Instead of trying to figure out a one-sided relationship where you are failing miserably at trying to change your body. What if you took a healthier approach? What if you started to acknowledge it for what is working? What if you recognized it for being your most loyal companion in this lifetime? What if you woke up every day and greeted your body from a new perspective?

One of the greatest things about a new relationship is that you have no frame of reference and no preconceived notions about who they are and they have no preconceived notions about who you are. There is no past baggage. So when you wake up with fresh eyes, and you say good morning body and begin to treat it with the excitement and anticipation you would have if you were going on a date with someone you really liked, you open the door to create a nurturing, loving, and alive relationship with your body.

Your body changes every day. When you acknowledge that your body loves to change, it will create an energy where you and your body get reacquainted with each other every day. What if your body could light you up every day? What if you could reset your metabolism? Reset your aging? Reset your pain? Reset?

Then take your body on a first date! Reset your relationship with a fresh perspective. Allow the excitement to create the energy of something new.

Be curious.

Ask questions.

Let go of any expectation or demand.

Ask it questions and get to know it. Be curious about what it likes and doesn't (and don't assume these preferences are permanent). Look at when it likes to eat, when it likes to move, what it likes to do for movement, who it likes to hang out with, what's nurturing for it, when it likes to sleep and how much. Pay attention to what it likes to do in its free time and what its style of communication is. It's always communicating with you. The question is, are you listening?

This isn't something you figure out right away, nor is it something you figure out just once. This is a daily practice of engaging. Developing a long-lasting, healthy relationship takes time, dedication, commitment, and persistence. You might get frustrated, and that's okay. A relationship takes two, and it is all about navigating, negotiating, requesting, and listening. Your body can ask and you can say no. Just like you can ask and your body can say no. This is about showing up to do the work. Go easy on yourself, it doesn't have to be perfect, there's no such thing.

A few years ago, I was in Europe on a six week long facilitating tour. I was facilitating 3-5 day workshops every week and traveling in between. The very last stop of the tour was in County Cork, Ireland.

My son was with me the entire time, from planes, to trains, to cars, and walking, my normal routine if I would have been alone was different. I wasn't getting as much exercise as I would have liked because he was pretty little.

The last couple days of teaching, I started to get some body sensations like I was about to get sick. So instead of just accepting my fate, I started to negotiate with my body and ask it questions.

I got that it was tired and it wanted desperately to be nurtured. So I negotiated with it. I said look: You have been amazing. You have been working hard for 6 straight weeks and I am so grateful. I would really like to not get sick, so what do you need?

Very clearly my body requested to have a massage and get it's bars run (Access Consciousness Bars). So I said, okay, let me make you a deal. I have two more days, on the third day, I promise to take the day off, get a massage and get my bars run.

It was that simple. I never got sick.

The book, *The Five Love Languages*, by Gary Chapman, may be helpful for you in communicating with your body. Its premise is that everyone has a different language in which they express love. Maybe you are someone who loves to receive gratitude verbally, or as the book calls it "words of affirmation." Therefore, one of your primary love languages is words of affirmation.

Now, if you are in a relationship with someone whose primary love language is quality time, and you keep telling them how much you love them but don't spend enough quality time with them, you could make yourself blue in the face with how much you express your love because they won't be able to hear you in the same way unless you start speaking their language.

Our bodies are the same way!

You and your body might have different love languages. If you don't acknowledge the difference, you might be talking at the same time without being dialed into the same radio station. It's hard to communicate when you're both talking on and listening to two completely different stations.

A big part of this entire challenge is the need to listen. Since the body doesn't speak the language of words, you have to be willing to be an expert at investigating your body's internal dialogue. And then acknowledge it for the language it speaks.

One of the ways to do this is to quiet the mind. Close your eyes, meditate if you meditate, and turn off any internal or external distractions. You can put one hand on your heart, one hand on your belly, or really anywhere your hands will take you deeper. Taking a few really slow, deep breaths with the eyes closed will allow you to connect inside. Then, with closed eyes, ask a question. And here's the trick: ask an engaging question, not a generic one.

> **What foods will make you happier after you're done eating them?**
>
> **What foods will make you feel sexy?**
>
> **What foods will make you feel wealthy?**

Those are engaging questions that you may not get the answers to right away. Remember that your body speaks in energy. It may flash a picture, you may experience a cool tingle on the back of your neck, or you might get goosebumps. Those are the moments in which your body is speaking to you loud and clear; it's just not in the form or the language you may have expected. That's why it's so important to develop a rapport with your body—to engage in leaning in, being curious, and then listening.

Like any good relationship, you don't need to agree with your body about everything. But for a healthy, long-lasting, nurturing relationship, you do have to listen and be good at listening.

Act like you and your body are always on a first date: ask questions and then be willing to listen…not just for the answer you want to hear, but listen for the actual dialogue of your body's own language. When you get where your body is functioning from—HOW and WHEN and WHERE and WHY—then you will begin to develop a line of communication with your body that even in the most challenging of circumstances will ring loud and clear.

When your body feels heard, just like when you feel heard, your body will contribute to you in ways that will surprise and delight you.

What are you waiting for?

Take your body on a first date!

Putting It Into Practice

- Grab a notebook and a pen. Put on some relaxing music, light a candle, set yourself up in a calming environment. Pour yourself a glass of wine or a glass of sparkling water.

- Go on a date with your body.

- Sit down with a notebook and write questions you would ask your body if you really wanted to get to know it—as if you were on a first date.

1. Treat your body with the curiosity of exploring something new. Below are some possible questions you could ask. Feel free to ask any questions that light you up! Remember, going on a date with your body should be FUN. Don't assume you know anything about your body. Remember, it is always changing and so are you, so start to engage as if you don't know.

2. What would you like to look like?

3. What would you change?

4. Do you feel heard?

5. What are some of the ways you're communicating with me and you feel like I'm not listening?

6. How can I better support you?

7. What are you asking for?

8. What's important to you?

9. What are your favorite foods? (The answers to this question will most likely be different than what you think.)

10. What foods have I been eating that don't work for you?

11. What foods will make you happier after you're done eating them?

12. What foods will make you feel sexy?

13. What foods will make you more money?

14. What foods would make you feel wealthy?

15. What foods would turn you on?

16. What foods would give you more energy?

You don't have to answer all the questions, but see which ones light you up and get you excited. Notice which questions are harder for you to answer. Notice how the questions make you feel, notice where in your body you feel them and also notice how your body is "talking" to you. Pay attention to goosebumps, cool breezes, energy in the palms, tingling, throat closing or opening, and so much more. Notice which questions you lean into and get excited to answer and which ones are harder to answer.

Remember, there is no right way or wrong way to do this. It is simply the willingness to become your own expert witness and embark on an adventure where you and your body create a healthy relationship where you both feel heard, seen, and understood.

17. Since we're in a relationship, what do you like about our relationship?

18. What don't you like about our relationship?

19. What would you change?

20. What are your deal breakers so when I do them, you act out?

Chapter 6
Wake up every day as if you just met your body!

"What I know for sure is this: The big secret in life is that there is no big secret... There's just you, this moment, and a choice."
—*Oprah*

When I was fresh out of my first year of grad school and living in Boulder, Colorado, I had just spent all my money on a two 1/2 month-long adventure traveling the world. I was tan for the first time in my life, had a shaved head, was free spirited and full of hope and possibilities. With less than $100 to my name, I was looking for a J.O.B. I had decided that the easiest choice with the most flexibility was to get a job bartending or waiting tables while I figured out my next move. I handed in 13+ resumes, and every manager looked me up and down and said, "We're full. We're not hiring."

I knew they were lying. I knew my shaved head didn't fit the tall blonde or petite brunette they were looking for. My shaved head made people uncomfortable. So, holding my head up high, in the heat of the sun on a hot summer day, I decided to go into one last restaurant. I pep talked myself—"You *got* this"—as I approached the restaurant. I walked in and asked to see the manager. An adorable, bubbly brunette said, "I'll be right back!"

From around the corner, this confident, hop-in-his-step man with piercing blue eyes, wearing a royal blue oxford and a yellow tie, was walking toward me. I did my best to hold my composure, but in the moment our eyes locked there was nothing to distract me. It was like everything slowed down and it felt like time stood still.

As he extended his hand to shake mine, I thought, "Oh, right, hand…"

As our hands shook, my entire body vibrated from the inside out. It was an experience I had never had before. We sat for what seemed like forever, with some of the time spent just staring into each other's eyes. I walked away from the exchange knowing I got the job, but there was way more happening beneath the surface.

That man became one of the loves of my life as well as the father of my son. We ultimately chose to go separate ways, but there were 8 amazing, head-over-heels, totally-in-love years.

I'm telling you this story to illustrate that there are these incredible spaces of time standing still. One of those captivating moments in time for me is when I met my son's father for the first time and we shook each other's hands. My entire body shook from the inside out. Our eyes locked and in those brief, few seconds I could perceive the pureness of our being. There were no walls, the insecurities were gone, and all that was left was the purity of possibilities.

During those moments, there are no preconceived notions, no judgments, no projections, no future tripping, no past reference points. It simply just *is*.

Of course I don't experience this with everyone I meet, but those that I do experience it with—women, men, new friendships, strangers, acquaintances, children—it's like a window where the dreamer in me, the romantic idealist that can perceive the gift in everyone, gets to dance for a very brief moment in time with another dreamer. It is one of my favorite things in the world.

What does this have to do with your relationship with your body?

Well, that spark you feel during those time-standing-still moments eventually fades. We inevitably start to pile on stories, expectations, projections, and judgments. And over time, that original space of newness and excitement fades. We no longer see the being but instead a mirror image of the judgments that we start to carry.

I believe that it's possible to regain the spark and the purity. In order to do that, we have to be very aware of the stories we have been telling ourselves about how we see ourselves.

Every day, when we wake up, look in the mirror, brush our teeth, get dressed, make our tea or coffee, the story of who we think we are and how the world sees us gets reinforced by our point of view of how we think we are seen.

The truth is that people see your gifts long before they see your judgments, but we ourselves see our judgments long before we see our gifts. In contrast, when you wake up in the morning and connect with your body as if you are meeting it for the very first time, you can begin to generate new neural pathways. Over time, the density of judgment can exit your body, leaving a window of time in which there is space, no judgment, no preconceived notions, no projections—just *space*. And in that space, anything is possible.

Imagine if you woke up every day and had the space to receive the gift your body came here to be.

It's hard for some of us to hear that there is truly NOTHING wrong with our bodies. Your body is not big boned. You don't have a slow metabolism. You didn't get the bad gene. You weren't born fat. Those thoughts all came in much later through conditioning based on your family, your environment, and your culture.

In my opinion, the best gift you can give yourself is to wake up and be happy. Wake up and be curious. Wake up and start to see you as if you were meeting you for the first time. What do you notice?

Someone once asked me,

"Who the heck wakes up every day and is completely different from the day before?"

Without hesitation and with an ear-to-ear grin I said "Me!" How could one *not* wake up a little different every day? The joy of having a body can be found when we are HAPPY with and in our bodies. **Change doesn't happen when we're sad, depressed, and judging our body.** Change gets created when we're happy, grateful, and appreciative. Those qualities create an energetic lightness that can change almost anything.

One of the keys, in fact, is **LIGHTNESS.** Have you ever tried to change something when you felt heavy, depressed, dark, or sad? Did it work? Imagine trying to create the future after waking up heavy. Imagine trying to create the future after waking up with preconceived notions of what is or isn't possible. The future gets created when we wake up curious, ask questions, and follow the energy. In my experience, forcing something into existence doesn't work.

Have you ever been so excited about a new adventure that everything in you buzzes with excitement? You dream of all the different ways this will work out? You dream of the future? I am a never-ending dreamer. From business to time with my son to adventures all over the world to all the lives that could change based on this idea of living a life of No Judgment, I am a never-ending dreamer.

The best weight loss advice I can give has only two parts:

1. No matter what, don't judge you or your choices.

2. BE HAPPY.

When I'm happy I make better life choices and better food choices. I workout, even if I don't want to, because I'm happy and I listen to what my body wants, which, most days, is to MOVE. I usually don't go to a gym because there's too much judgment in a gym. So I get outside...I ski, I bike, I hike up a mountain, I go for a run, I connect to nature. Or I put music on in my living room and dance. Or I get my butt to a hot yoga or hot pilates class. It all depends on how I'm feeling. But whatever it is, I MOVE.

I don't move to look good (that's just a benefit). I move because movement changes my energy; it invoragtes me, it stabilizes my mood, it dissipates any energy I'm holding onto that I need to let go of. Bodies need to move energy. They need to let go, change temperature, sweat, and so much more. If you're not big on movement, start to ask, "Body, how would you like to move your energy today?"

Ask...and then listen.

Remember, your body won't tell you in words, but it will tell you in energy. When you wake up, be curious about what's possible. Wake up and ask a question. Open the door to something different by re-introducing yourself to your body. Express gratitude for it and look at it with childlike curiosity. Just like you, your body changes its mind as much, if not more, than you. It also changes its shape, weight, likes, and dislikes.

Just like you, it changes. So what worked for you and your body last month or last year may not have the same effect now. Your body entirely regenerates itself every 7 years. Every second, in fact, *10,000* cells die and *10,000* new cells are born. That means, in a 24-hour period, 864 million new cells regenerate in the body. So, every single day, you have the chance to reprogram 864 million new cells and give them the energy of the future.

Change is easy. Resisting change is hard.

Most people have decided that if change occurs they will lose something. What I've found is that in the wake of change, the only thing we lose is our limitations and all the things that keep us stuck. Most of us have worked very hard to maintain our limitations. What if you were willing to wake up everyday as if you didn't have any limitations?

Every morning when you wake up, you're different. Your body is different. **The body changes everyday. You change everyday.**

Both of you are different everyday, so it's time to start relating to your body differently and allow your body to relate to you differently. If you've been relating to your body from the space of who it was yesterday, last month, or last year, it's time to change how you're relating to it.

When you wake up everyday and decide to relate to your body from a place of having met for the first time, like a first date, you begin to ask questions and be curious about your body. It's new, it's exciting, and it might have new information for you today.

When you wake up with a sense of wonder, the body has space to relax. When you don't project, reject, or decide what the body needs to look like, there is a space where you give the body permission to create itself. For me, that sense of space means that if you're having a bad day it's not the end of the world.

During times that I have been in the thick of my own self-judgment and criticism, I rampantly go down the rabbit hole of internal conflict and turmoil. If I would overeat, even by just a bite or two, I would decide it was the end of the world. Sometimes I'd spend the next several hours binge eating, stuffing my face, beating me up, and then laying in a food coma surrounded by a painful, judgmental fog.

It was a very vicious cycle, one where I never gave myself permission to have any room for error. Can you imagine what it would be like if you were cranky or pissed off about something that you genuinely have permission to be cranky or pissed off about and your body tells you that you don't have permission to be upset? You'd be like, "Screw you!" Well, guess what? The body *also* gets cranky. As a result, it might retain water, create pain or tension, or gain weight.

Give your body permission to be cranky when it's having a cranky moment! And stop going into the need to fix it. Because when you don't make your body (or you) wrong for its changes, then it can change even quicker in a way that works for you.

Here's an example: At one point while I was writing this book, I got really sick. Sick in a way I don't think I had ever been sick before. I had been asking for a few specific things to change with me, and I didn't expect to get sick. But sick was the way my body needed to be at that time, and allowing it to be sick gave it permission to change something that I had been needing to change for most of my life.

It was painful being sick like that. I could barely walk, I certainly couldn't exercise, and I could barely eat. I spent a few days shaking in bed under the covers, going from hot and sweaty to cold and freezing. It took every ounce of strength I could find just to walk to the bathroom. I had to muster up all my energy just to get on the phone with clients. I had to cancel a few days of calls, which rarely ever happens and I showed up on one of my telecalls barely able to talk.

Ultimately, I recovered. After giving my body permission to be sick, I had more clarity and more space for the change I had been asking for. The point is, during its period of sickness my body was changing. And it NEEDED the space to change. It needed to rest, sleep, not eat much. It needed to sweat and shake, It didn't need me up in its business getting mad, frustrated, or upset.

So I rested. I slept. I thanked my body for what it was going through. I wasn't mad. I wasn't antsy. I wasn't upset. I was grateful. I didn't freak out. I didn't stress about my health or the fact I wasn't working.

It was probably the first time in my adult life that I gave myself permission to ENJOY the rest. To enjoy the change, to just ALLOW it. When you allow the body to do what it needs to do, it is changing energy. It changes through all sorts of methods and means. Don't judge it. Judging it stops the momentum of change. You don't have to like it, but relax, let go, and just stop judging it. Let your body do its thing. When you get use to the idea that it is changing FOR YOU, you will begin to relax,

Here's another example: A few years ago, I was looking at my body, and the skin above my knees looked old. It was kind of freaky. It was like I had never seen that skin before, and I thought, "Oh crap! I'm aging!" And then I stopped myself and used my own advice. I asked, "Body, what are you doing?" The energetic response I got back was "I'm changing." I said, "Ok, cool. Is there anything you need from me?" What I got back was "Relax and let us change." I said, "Ok."

The next day I was on a radio show, and in the middle of talking I looked down at my knees and the skin was back to normal. Again, kind of freaky. I thought, "Holy crap, body! You are so amazing! Thank you for showing me what's possible."

These examples are so telling. When we don't conclude or go into wrongness about the body's changes, then its ability to be resilient and bounce back can just occur, seemingly like a miracle. Your body is a miracle. When given permission to do whatever it needs, it will surprise you, show you something more amazing than you thought possible. You just have to be in allowance, have gratitude, and know that it has your back. When you give your body permission to have a bad day, it knows you trust it more. When your body trusts that you won't freak out, it can change quicker.

There's nothing worse than being in a relationship where the other person doesn't trust you.

When your body feels like you trust it, it can relax and so can you. In contrast, every time your body does something that might not work for you and you go into the wrongness—creating a conclusion that you're getting fat or struggling with your body—you are treating your body as if it doesn't have permission to change, have a day of rest, or choose something different.

This may sound crazy, but when you don't trust your body, when you don't relax into knowing it is always doing its best to take care of you, then you begin to create an environment and an experience where you don't feel safe in your own body. And when you don't feel safe you will invent stories about what's going on that isn't actually true. When our safety is threatened (real or imagined) our reptilian brain takes over and we go into fight, flight, fawn, or freeze.

> *"The most well-known responses to trauma are the fight, flight, or freeze responses. However, there is a fourth possible response, the so-called fawn response. Flight includes running or fleeing the situation, fight is to become aggressive, and freeze is to literally become incapable of moving or making a choice. The fawn response, often developed in childhood trauma, involves immediately moving to try to please a person to avoid any conflict."*
> —*Sherry Gaba LCSW*

So what does this have to do with your body and the weight you so desire to lose? When there are hidden bouts of trauma stuck in the body, you will do whatever you can to try to create safety. This underlying hidden subconscious feeling of not being safe (even if you are) can drastically impact one's ability to effectively change weight. Especially if the weight was created to overcome a trauma that involved not feeling safe. When I was 17 my brother, in a fit of rage, threatened to take my life. I got free and processed that trauma, but what I didn't process until recently, was what happened after that.

My mother came home to cop cars in her driveway. She was a single mom of 4 kids who also had a career that depended on her reputation. When she came home to the scene that ensued in her driveway, her fight, flight, freeze, or fawn responses were activated and in a panic, my mother lost it.

Ultimately, I no longer felt safe in my own home and moved in with my best friend and her family. I spent the summer feeling safe, loved, and cared for. But then it came time to go back to school and I needed to move back home.

I didn't realize it, but I felt so unsafe. That year, which was my senior year in high school, I gained 20 pounds. My need to feel safe was compromised, and therefore my body's ability to cope under extreme duress, led to me gaining weight, which began an almost 20 year cycle of ups and downs with my weight, feeling unsafe, and the inability to cope with stress in my body.

When it comes to wanting to lose weight, if your safety has been compromised in your own home, then you may have unconsciously or subconsciously created behaviors or belief patterns that attempt to satiate your need to feel safe. Your body may have compromised something in order to protect you. And this could have led to a lifelong struggle with your weight.

If you truly have problems, then the work is to get curious. Don't assume you have a problem, instead find out what's hiding underneath? What's the cause of you feeling unsafe, or insecure, or not enough. If you truly can't lose, ask: what's underneath the desire to lose weight? And at what point did you decide you couldn't lose weight? At what point did you give up your ability to react and respond in a healthy way when it comes to food and your body?

When did you start to feel unsafe in your own body? When you begin to acknowledge the root triggers from an emotional and energetic standpoint then everything can change. This isn't about recreating the story and re-traumatizing yourself. This is about energetically identifying what's keeping you from the change you truly desire. When you let go of the energy of it, then your body can do what it does best, which is to naturally heal itself. Most of our attempts to control our weight come from this deep innate ache inside to feel safe. It's hard to feel happy and free when you intrinsically don't feel safe.

The good news is it's not your fault. The good news is, you're not as screwed up as you think you are. The good news is, your body was born to heal and it can heal quickly. Part of the process of healing is to resource yourself with energies that make you come alive. Start fresh, see yourself through the eyes of someone who utterly and completely adores you. Give yourself the same grace and kindness you give others. You want the people you love and adore to be happy, so start by choosing to be happy with yourself first.

Find those small ways everyday to be grateful for what you do have, for what your body can do, and for all the ways it's been there for you no matter what.

Putting It Into Practice

Here's a morning ritual you can try:

When you first open your eyes, while still laying in bed, put one hand on your belly, one hand on your heart, and take a few deep breaths. Thank your body for being so amazing and then ask some questions:

What did you change last night?

What can I contribute to the change?

What would you like to create today?

And then take another moment to truly thank your body. Thank it for taking such good care of you. Imagine waking up next to your intimate other and in the morning they ask, "How did I get so lucky to be with you?" Imagine saying *that* to your body. Doesn't that sound like a great way to wake up?

Then think of all 864 million new cells in your body and ask them to energetically calibrate to the future—to health, to wealth, to healing, and to anything and everything else you are creating.

Think about it as developing an amazing relationship with your body. And we know that a few key components of a healthy relationship are communication, allowance, and gratitude. Not judgment, ridicule, and lack.

No one can tell you how to do a relationship.

After you have calibrated, then ask the body to turn on the health of all its cells. Remember that when you meet someone for the first time, there are NO reference points to go back to. No past experiences. It is new. It is now. If you treat your body like that everyday, imagine the kind of life you could live…one with kindness, presence, gratitude, and so much more.

One of the many things that amazed me about this process was that **once I truly got out of judgment I had so much space to create, to dream, to imagine, to implement, and to play.** And as long as I was creating, there was no time or space to allow judgment to impede the forward momentum. If you want to explore this morning routine a little more, grab your notebook and at the top of the page write:

Body, what would you like to create today?

What can I contribute to you?

Write down everything you get. Don't filter it. Don't judge it. Don't squash it. Just like a kid full of dreams and possibilities, your body just wants to be heard. So give it the space to be heard. The more you do this, the more you will get to know your body, it's desires, wishes, and changes and in turn you will get to know you too.

Chapter 7
Be curious and ask questions! The Power of a Question

"This is the place where problems end and creation begins"
—*Katherine McIntosh*

Do you change a lot? Do you change your mind all the time? Do you change what you desire to create from day to day? If you answered yes, then chances are your body changes just as much as you do.

Your body changes constantly. So, considering that it is changing all the time, imagine what it would be like if you asked your body questions instead of jumping to conclusions about what's wrong with it? Imagine asking questions instead of trying to figure out the perfect fix.

Questions always create greater.

"The reality you create is based on the questions you ask."
—Dr. Dain Heer

So if you want a greater reality with your body, then start asking questions that light you up. Start asking questions that make you happy when you ask them. Ask questions from a place of gratitude, not from a place of judgment.

So instead of asking: How do I lose weight? (I don't think that makes anyone happy) or what's wrong with me that I can't lose weight? Ask: What energies would my body like to play with today? What foods would make my body feel alive? What can I wear that would make me feel amazing?

Think about this in terms of a relationship. What would it create if you said to your sweet amazing husband: why didn't you take the garbage out? That's obviously a question from judgment. But if you said, hey lover, I'm so grateful for how much you do to keep the house and the family alive, would you mind taking the garbage out for me?

You'd probably get a much different response. The body is the same way. No one likes to be told what to do, including your body. It likes and responds to questions. It doesn't like to be told; it likes to be asked. Your body is not a problem to be solved. Your body is a possibility to create with. So start treating it like a possibility and not a problem.

Let me reiterate that most diets are based on what worked for someone else. Because it worked once, they offered it to other people. But certain things work for certain bodies while other things don't. A diet is a set plan. It is not a question. So start to get curious about all the things that make you happy when you look at it. What foods, movements, people, energies, clothes make you happy? Find out and do more of that. Get curious about certain foods, and diet possibilities and instead of adopting the whole plan find out what about the plan works for you. Here's one question that could start to open up a possibility between you and your body:

What would work for my body?

Anything with a fixed plan doesn't leave room for questions. For example, when I started my business of traveling around the world doing what I love, I had no idea how to run a business based on trusting my knowing. Even though I had always found ways to be successful, I still paid tens of thousands of dollars to business coaches. The only problem was, their advice never worked for me.

I knew their advice didn't work for me. I was aware that *I knew something they didn't know*, but that was not something I was willing to look at. I actually *knew* and didn't need to pay people to show me that I knew. I just didn't trust myself yet. So I ended up paying a lot of money to people so I could discover that I actually knew more than they did about what was required for the businesses and future I wanted to create.

When I implemented their advice, it didn't work, and then I got caught up in trying to fix the problems I created by following other people's advice. It took me a long time to get back to trusting me and following what lights me up. I still have a long way to go and a lot to learn, but the difference is I now take people's advice and filter it through: will this work for me? Will this work for the future I desire to create? Will this work for the business? What about this will work? And what about this won't work? Like many of us, I've had some very expensive lessons in life.

The same thing happens with people and their bodies—not trusting that they actually know what's best. Most people have decided they don't know what works. They get confused because there are so many conflicting messages and the messages change all the time. So when they try something and it doesn't work, they get frustrated and decide there's something wrong with them. That is the biggest mistake we can make: deciding that there is something wrong with us, instead of discovering there is something wrong with this system. The truth is: there is nothing wrong with you. When you come from that perspective, then you are in charge of your healing, transformation, and change.

When you are disempowered and decide it's hard to change something, you make someone else the expert of you. But the truth is: YOU are the EXPERT. When you empower yourself to be the expert of your own body, to investigate, get curious, experiment, and explore, then you can discover what works for you. When you are empowered, you are willing to ask yourself: what would work for your body, your environment, your situation. When you are empowered, you are willing to experiment and you're not afraid of getting it wrong.

Most people haven't yet had long-term success with losing weight, getting fit, staying healthy, and discovering what works for them. What actually works isn't something that's been taught mainstream.

What works is to ask questions, be curious, and stop treating your body like it's something to feed, sleep, and poop. Your body is not something you train. It isn't a problem to be solved. It's a possibility to explore. If you want to have communion and peace with your body, within a space of gratitude, you have to be willing to explore the possibilities of it.

As a parent, I can take advice and educate myself about parenting, but no one can tell me how to parent. I trust my knowing when it comes to raising my son. It's the same with your body. No one can tell you how to be with your body. Ultimately, you know. You have always known.

When you take other people's advice as if they know more than you do, you give up trusting you. Not trusting you is very costly. No one can tell you about your body. They can invite you, ask you, and give you information, but only you KNOW.

Years ago in the midst of my first marriage. I was sick. Like really sick. After 9 months of tests, doctors, diagnosis's, pills, and experiments, no one could figure out what was wrong with me.

I was falling apart and in a fit of desperation a woman invited me to have a session with her. I had no idea what she did, but I walked into her office fully clothed and laid on a massage table. She put one hand on my sacrum, and one hand on my belly and she started to ask me what my body knows.

She asked what my gut was telling me. And it was the first time I was able to admit that my marriage wasn't working, I was miserable, and was working 100 hour weeks to avoid the truth that my marriage was an awful mess.

In all the 9 months of doctors visits, hospitals, tests, and explorations, not one person asked me what my body knew. Not one person inquired about what was going on in my life.

Everyone wanted to treat the symptom, but no one looked at what was causing the symptom in the first place...

Until that fateful session.

It was the first time in over 9 months I had immediate physical relief because she was willing to explore what was causing the symptom. And the truth was: my body had the answers. It was an eye opening experience and one that led me down a path to dive into the mind, body, healing connection.

It was the beginning of me knowing i wanted to spend the rest of my life working with the mind body connection.

The Moment I Knew that the Body Knows

One cold winter evening after a very satisfying workout and then a soak in the hot springs, I was in the locker room getting dressed and saw this woman with this long, luscious hair across the room. She was drinking some kind of green drink. At that moment, it was like a force greater than me, possessed me. I jumped up half naked and ran over to her. "What is that??" I asked. "Whatever it is, I need it!"

A few days prior, I was getting an itch to amp up my health. I was feeling lethargic and sluggish. I was going through a lot of change, and I knew my body needed a boost. I kept getting this "green energy" but I didn't know what that meant, so I said to my body, "Whatever that energy is, let's pull it in and can you please make it really obvious when we find it?"

Well, that moment in the locker room, it was obvious and my body took over before I knew what to do with myself, until I realized I was half naked having a conversation with a mere stranger. She said she'll never forget that moment. We had a good laugh, she told me about the drink, it gave me the boost I needed, and from that moment on we became good friends.

The point is, the body knows. You just have to invite it to be an active participant in the creation of your life. Include it. Ask it questions. Give it jobs.

I like to give my body the jobs of finding the best food, eating at the best restaurants, and making travel around the world really easy. I give it a job, and then I get out of the freaking way. I think this has given me the capacity to travel in total ease. While traveling I often get things for free—like upgrades, meals, and even bottles of wine—because I allow my body to be in charge.

I ask my body to do things for me all the time.

When you engage with your body in that way—trusting it, asking it questions, giving it a job and getting out of its way—you invite it to engage with the world. And when you allow your body to be the living, breathing, incredible example of possibilities that it came here to be, then life gets easier.

What kinds of things do our bodies like? Most bodies on the planet love to be lusted after. They love the energy of being turned on—turned on by nature, turned on by creativity, turned on by connection, good food, great company, good art, fascinating music. It's like a painter in the moment...so tapped into the creative, generative energies that he forgets to eat and sleep. He is just purely in the moment; the world disappears and yet everything is available to him in that moment. He is connected, alive, invigorated, and inspired. There is no room for judgment in those turned on moments.

When you allow your body not to cut itself off to the generative energies, it becomes a walking, talking generator of aliveness that attracts possibilities. When you are turned onto life, you are like a giddy kid, tapped into a totally different universe where anything is possible.

This sense of curiosity, wonderment, and adventure opens a door to the universe being able to contribute to you.

When you are in this energy, there is no room for judgment. Judgment cannot exist simultaneously when you are tapped into the aliveness, to the curiosity, and to the sense of adventure.

I experienced many moments of feeling that tapped in on my first overseas trip to a non-English speaking country: Barcelona (still one of my favorite cities in the world). I remember wandering the cobblestone streets, seeing the architecture, the colors, listening to the sounds, the incantation of chatter that sounded more like birds singing—it was all so fascinating that I would forget to eat. It took my breath away, and I would get completely lost in the moment. Interestingly, I think I came back from that trip 10 pounds lighter.

When we function from curiosity and become a question, it feels light and easy. The other path is hardness, harshness, and force. And no one likes to be forced. Whenever we are forced to do something, most of us get upset, grumpy, and frustrated.

When you're grumpy or in a bad mood and your significant other clearly sees you're in a bad mood, it's really tough when they keep asking, "What's wrong with you? Why are you so grumpy? Why are you in a bad mood?"

It's unkind to not be in allowance of the range of emotions that we go through on a daily basis. This comes up a lot for me with raising a child. Part of my challenge as a parent is that my son experiences every emotion under the sun in any given second. It's not kind if I teach him that he isn't allowed to experience all the changes of life. Instead, I'll ask him, "What's up? What do you need? What do you know?" What if we extended this same level of kindness and allowance to our ever changing bodies? When the body gets grumpy, irritable, or is in pain, it's usually because it's trying to change something. It's not trying to upset you, frustrate you, or make your life harder. So go easy on it. It's trying to contribute to you. Ask it: What's up? What do you need? What do you know? What are you trying to change? It will tell you if you listen.

Your Body Has Your Back

When you are experiencing change, your body will change to support you. Your body desires to change to contribute to you. Your body has your back. If it didn't have your back, you'd probably be dead. You wouldn't be here...your body would've checked out a long time ago.

When you ask your body a question and it answers in energy, often the body is responding in a way we believe we can't hear. But it's not that you can't hear the body; it's that you've *decided* you don't understand it.

So, be patient. Listen. Let go of all preconceived notions of what this needs to look like and just let it be. The body is speaking to you in energy all day long, like the intuitive hit to get your oil changed or have your car checked before hitting the road. It's the intuitive hit to call a friend you haven't spoken to in a long time and they respond by saying, "I was just thinking about you." There are so many subtle ways in which the body communicates, but so often, because it rarely feels like a brick over the head, we think the body isn't communicating.

So much of this book is about asking questions and being open to receiving the energy. If you truly want to have a body and life that continues to get greater with time, then start asking as many questions as you can. Ask them from curiosity and gratitude, and be willing to listen for the answer. Be patient. Remember, this is an adventure, not a destination to be right. A true question doesn't always have an immediate answer, but it will have an immediate energy. One of my favorite questions to ask when I don't know what question to ask is:

Body, what question can I ask that will change all of this?

Usually I get an energy in response. And then that energy gifts me an awareness, the whisper of the change I was looking for. Sometimes that whisper is just a simple knowing. When it comes to the body, there are no answers. There are only moments in time that work, and then it changes. We are always changing, and if we are truly going to have a body we are HAPPY with then it is about being curious.

The next time you are in search of an answer that comes in the form of a conclusion, try asking, **Body, what question can I ask that will change this?**

Personally, whenever I come to the conclusion that I need to lose weight, I am not as happy and I tend to eat more. Then my body gains weight and life gets a little harder. Whenever this happens, Instead of making the demand to lose weight or get fitter, I ask: what choice can I make that would make me happier today?

When I am living my life, creating, playing outside, and connecting, I ask questions like, "Body, what would make you happy? Body, what foods would make you feel sexy? Body, what would give you more energy? What would contribute to having more confidence?" When I ask those kinds of questions there is always a lightness. I may not have or know the answer, but the energy I receive is the gift that creates something different. Never once in asking those questions has it ever answered back with the need to go on a diet.

There is no right way or wrong way; there is only choice, question, possibility, and contribution.

Everything that occurs in our lives is a contribution, even if it comes in the form of a hard-knock lesson. The key is not to judge you or what transpires so that you can be open to receive the gift that is occurring even if you can't see it in the moment.

If you don't see it as a problem, it can always turn into a possibility.

This same principle applies if you are in pain. Pain is the body's way of turning up the volume to get your attention about something you aren't changing or choosing. So ask, **"Body, what do you want me to know? What are you facilitating me toward?"**

Questions always empower. Pain is simply the body's attempt to get your attention. So instead of making the pain wrong, ask a question, get curious. Be there when it responds, just like you would be there for your child when they are in pain. When you ask a question, you eliminate the need to hide your insecurities. Not knowing creates a new beginning.

When you go on a first date, do you know how it's going to turn out before you go? Not necessarily. You have to be curious and present and in constant question, and you want your date to be curious about you… that's what makes a great date.

Putting It Into Practice

If you would like to start using questions to see how that could change your body, here are a few you can begin to play with. Your invitation is to ask these questions and then begin to notice all the different ways in which your body responds. Again, it might be goosebumps, a lightness in your chest, tingling in your palms, a hot flash, a nose flair, a yawn, a tear, a head rush. Pay attention, this is how your body is communicating to you. The more you show it that you truly are listening, the more it will communicate to you in ways that work for you and it will start to diminish the ways in which it thinks it needs to scream at you to get your attention.

> **What foods would light you up today, body?**
>
> **What is your favorite way to play?**
>
> **What's right about this I'm not getting?**
>
> **What size of sexy would you like to be?**
>
> **What would give you more energy today?**
>
> **What can I contribute to you today?**
>
> **What are you aware of?**
>
> **What would you like to say today?**
>
> **What would you like to do to move your body today?**
>
> **What clothes would make you feel like a million bucks today?**
>
> **Is there something that you would like to do that would create more in every area of our life together?**

What are some foods that would inspire you to create a greater life?

There are no stupid questions. So ask away. You can come up with any question you want. **The power of a question is to create the space for awareness** rather than come to a conclusion. There have been many times where I thought I was asking a question that allowed for possibilities, but then I would conclude that the answer was a permanent solution. **The body changes as much as you change your mind about everything.** So be in question always. Follow your knowing every day. It will change from moment to moment. When you get the hit to follow your awareness, do it. If it no longer feels like it's working, just continue to be in question.

Remember, this is an experiment. You can't become an expert ballerina by taking one ballet class. Show up. Show up every day. Let yourself fall. Get back up and keep going. You got this! You're a rockstar.

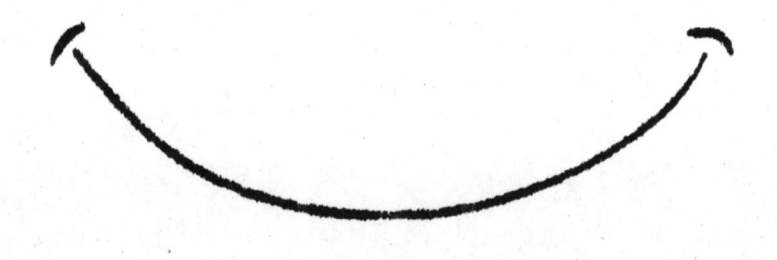

Chapter 8
Have gratitude for what your body can do!

"I finally realized that being grateful to my body was key to giving more love to myself."
—**Oprah**

Having gratitude for your body can lead to finding energy and strength you didn't know you had. There I was half-way up the mountain, huffing and puffing and somewhat grunting. I was 2+ hours into a hike with no water and no food. I had left the house to go for a quick stroll in the mountains, which at the time was right outside my back door. As I left, I thought, "I'll just go for a bit."

But I was pumping adrenaline from an argument with my sister who was visiting. In the heat of a hot summer day, I became possessed. I kept going and going and going, and pretty soon I realized that I was going to the top, no matter what. At this time in my life, climbing up mountains that normally take 4-5 hours was not something I did on a regular basis.

My body was tired, but I just kept having gratitude for the fact that 2+ hours in I was still going. I kept asking, "Body, what are you capable of that I'm not letting you choose." It was amazing: Everytime I asked that question, I'd get a burst of energy and a fire in my belly to keep going. When I started to get lethargic, when I felt I needed water, when my muscles were fatigued, I asked and that ask gave me so much energy.

Notice how asking a question gave me that energy. I didn't go into conclusion or decide anything; I kept asking questions, and each time I did a space opened up and I kept going. On that hike, it was like there was no "can't" in my universe. Instead: "What are you capable of?" was in my universe. When we say "can't," we are correct, but when we say "can," we are also correct, no matter what it takes. A question allows the "I can" to emerge...as if by magic, not by force.

I firmly believe that we need to stop focusing on what we can't do. Instead, start focusing on what you *can* do. Your body will surprise you if you stop telling it what it can't do. No one likes to be told what they can and can't do. Your body is the same way. Give it some credit and allow it to show up for you.

I had the experience in college of learning to allow my body to show up for me. I almost played soccer for the university, but the coach was extremely intense. She looked at me and said, "If you want on this team, you're going to have to eat, breathe, and sleep soccer." It was at that moment that a bright-eyed midwestern girl, who found herself in Montana and in the mountains, realized she wanted to explore and have an adventure beyond soccer, beyond what she had ever chosen before.

That was the beginning of me exploring a whole new world. One day, my good friend Sam, who was a mountain biking maniac from Hawaii, asked me to go biking with him. He called me "Katrine," which I loved, and his enthusiasm and love for the sport was infectious. He was one of those crazy people who could ride up the side of the mountain without thinking about it, doing things no one else would dare to do, and then have the biggest smile on his face when he came back down.

So, on this fateful spring day, at Sam's request, I pulled out my Trek bike. It was brand new but had no shock absorbers—a basic bike, definitely not built to ride down a mountain, especially in mountain biking country. We got to the top, he looked at me with a big grin, and said, "Follow me."

So I did. And holy *CRAP*. I was laughing, freaking out, and holding on for dear life.

At some points there were jumps that Sam would launch off of. There was no way in hell I was jumping, so I rode through them as best I could using my breaks. I held on for dear life. I made every face you could make...and kept going. I had a few close calls, but never once fell. I was using my brakes so much that they started to make a squeaking sound. Sam looked behind and saw me and said, "HOLY SHIT, Katrine, what are you doing?!"

I looked at him with these innocent eyes and smiled and said, "Following you." He looked at me both with disbelief and with a giant grin on his face. And that was the beginning of my mountain biking love affair.

The point is, I didn't have any idea what I was capable of. I didn't tell myself I couldn't. I didn't overthink it. I just kept going. And every time I did, I surprised myself. As long as I wasn't telling myself "I can't,"

I was physically capable of way more than I ever thought possible. After that experience, I went to the bike shop and special ordered my first mountain bike.

Our bodies are capable of so much more than we give them credit for. And we don't have to think about it like mind over matter; it can just be a question. **What is your body capable of that you never considered?**

Still, it took me a long time to realize how much I continued to judge my body. Even as I developed a passion for mountain biking and fitness, I always had this secret judgment: I always thought my legs were too big. Without any kindness, I referred to them as "tree trunks". For years, I was never able to be grateful for my legs. In fact, I spent probably 20 years obsessing over the backs of my legs, convinced I had cellulite for days. Notice how there was no gratitude, only judgment. It is impossible to have gratitude and judge yourself at the same time.

I started the No Judgment Diet out of sheer desperation, when all those years of secretly judging myself finally caught up to me. As I stood in the middle of my hallway, my jeans half way up my thighs—sweating, swearing, with tears running down my face—I had completely lost myself in the self-torture of judgment. I forgot I had a son. I forgot that I had created this beautiful life. I couldn't see myself; I couldn't have gratitude for myself. I couldn't see the good or the blessings in my life.

At that moment, I knew I had to change. And I knew I couldn't wait another day, couldn't put off living another day. It hit me like a ton of bricks. I had lived my whole freaking life in judgment. In hate. In disgust. And that took me out of living. Enough was enough. *Now* was the time.

As I stood there and saw my son beaming gratitude at me, I picked him up and just held him with all my might. Thanking him for the gift he was. Thanking him for no judgment. And so it began. I started to look at myself in the mirror and forced myself to find things to be grateful for.

> *"Gratitude is the key to producing miracles."*
> —*Gary Douglas*

This part of my journey with my body—forcing myself to find things about my body to be grateful for—was one of the hardest to put myself through. There were days I wanted to scream and cry, days that even trying to find one thing about my body to be grateful for felt like an impossibility.

But day after day, I'd get in front of the mirror, strip down naked, and actually look at my body with curious eyes. Could I see myself the way others had for years? Throughout my adult life, people had complimented me and my body, told me how beautiful I was, how sexy, athletic, strong, determined. But I couldn't hear any of it. For 20 years I had convinced myself that everyone was lying to me. I always thought to myself, "I am not beautiful. I am not sexy. Heck, I am not even athletic. Can't you see my flaws?"

Their compliments did not match the judgments I had of myself, so I would reject them. Sometimes I couldn't even *hear* the compliment because I was so immersed and self-absorbed in my own little judgmental pity party. I couldn't hear anything that didn't match my judgment of myself.

For years, my second husband and the father of my son heard me complain about my appearance. He witnessed the nights I missed attending an event because I would sit in my closet in tears telling him I wasn't pretty enough, skinny enough, beautiful enough.

The Disease of Judgment

> *"Health and wellness can be as infectious as disease."*
> —Katherine McIntosh

This disease I had was debilitating. I look back on it in disbelief. And sadly, this epidemic of body judgment is so widespread. It hits people of all shapes and sizes. I hope this book invites people to see that if I can come out of this judgmental hell hole and create a life that truly fuels me and fills me up, then anyone can do it.

The trick is to use tools and resources, find support, get out of your own way, and, most of all, practice gratitude. Choosing to lose weight will not make you happy, but choosing to be happy can help you change your body in miraculous ways! Choosing no judgment allows you to shed more weight than you can imagine. Judgments weigh a lot. They can weigh down our spirit, our sanity, our joy, and our desire to live.

There I was standing in my hallway, jeans around my thighs, for the first time trying to find things about my body to be grateful for. With my son in my arms, I looked at this precious being and realized there wasn't one single inch of him I would judge. I took a long, deep breath and then I looked at myself. I scanned my body up and down, and deep pain and sadness emerged. For 20 years I had been judging my body. I was an expert at self-hatred, self-judgment, and self-ridicule. At that moment, for the first time ever, I truly apologized to my body and asked for forgiveness. "Please forgive me," I said, "for being the most evil hate monger in the world." And as I stood there with tears streaming down my face, I found a glimmer of hope.

"Oh!" I thought. "My eyes! I have beautiful, sparkling, light-up-the-world-when-I-smile eyes." After a few seconds, more gratitude showed up: "Oh! I have a great smile. That smile has made thousands of people break out into a spontaneous smile." Then another piece of gratitude emerged: "I like my freckles. I have always liked my freckles."

That was the beginning of a journey that took me from disdain for my appearance to one of gratitude. It took several months, but eventually I could look at my legs and instead of judging them I started to have gratitude for all the goals they scored in soccer, all the miles they ran, mountains they climbed, ski hills they skied down, countries and streets they walked through. Once I adopted gratitude as a way of living with my body, not only did my body begin to morph and change, but my life began to morph and change as well.

I started to see possibilities that before seemed impossible. I started to have a completely different outlook on life. The more I paid attention to all the places in my life that were working, I no longer had time to judge me. It was like my train had finally been filled with steam, instead of lumps of coal, and there was no stopping me. As the energy in my body shifted, I felt sexier. My muscle tone came back without me having to work out. Laughter gave me abs, and there was this freedom in creating my life as a new mom with a new outlook on life. It was the first time ever, I saw a glimmer of hope that it could be possible that I could be happy in my own body...

The year I went on the No Judgment Diet, I didn't lose a lot of weight, but my body went from a size 8/10 to a 4/6. My clothes fit differently. I was eating everything that I loved and I no longer had a desire to binge, sneak food, obsess about what to eat and what not to eat. Because my energy shifted, my focus also shifted. Instead of pouring all my energy into my body to try to change it, I was pouring all my energy into my new business. I started a business when my son was 5 months old, I had less than $1,000 to my name, and in 10 months I had crossed the $100,000 mark doing what I LOVED! I couldn't believe it. It was definitely a "pinch me" moment and a huge wake up call. If I could do this, I wondered how many women were out there struggling with their body weight, image, and food. I wondered how many women would radically transform their lives if they knew that changing their body was possible?

I tell my story because it reveals to me how much our lives can change when we stop judging our bodies. I never thought I could make a 6+ figure income doing what I love. I never thought I'd be able to get paid for doing energy work. And yet I had always dreamed of having a practice that invited people to wake up to their body's own healing capacities. But I had to stop judging my own body before that practice became possible.

The body can heal itself and does almost every day.

Remember that, every 24 hours, our bodies create 864 million new cells. That's like a whole new reality every 24 hours if you're willing to have gratitude, be curious, and allow the body to do what it was designed to do…heal itself. **If we start to choose gratitude, the new cells coming into your body every second can take on a different energy and not only regenerate the body but rejuvenate it as well.**

Does your body have the capacity to change as quickly as you do?

We often conclude that it takes forever to change the body—that it's hard to lose weight, and challenging to decrease the pain that may be present in the body. Yet in my 20+ years of working with the energy of a body, I have seen miracles. The miracles happen when we let go of any preconceived notion of what is or isn't possible.

I believe that our bodies are much quicker than we've given them credit for. What if your body can change something instantaneously? What if you allowed for the change to actualize? Be patient—if you conclude that your body isn't changing, then it will stop the change it was choosing.

Gratitude is the highest vibration there is.

> *"Gratitude changes everything. Judgment changes nothing."*
> —*Dr. Dain Heer*

I believe that gratitude is higher than love. As someone who once associated love with abuse, I know that love can be confusing. But gratitude has no gray area to it. You cannot fake gratitude. It just is. There is no double meaning. And when you choose to be grateful for you, for your body, and for everything around you, you change the molecules in your body, which in turn can change your appearance.

I didn't believe it was possible to change your appearance by changing your judgments, until one day, when I was standing in front of the mirror feeling forlorn because of the cellulite on the backs of my thighs.

There I was, standing in front of the mirror and trying to let go of the judgments I had about the cellulite on the backs of my legs. And as I began to let go of the judgments, I started to have gratitude for that area. I started thanking my body for not giving up on me, for not hating me for 20 years of judgment and ridicule.

Then, all of the sudden, the cellulite started to diminish. I couldn't believe it! At first, I was convinced I was crazy. There is NO WAY that is possible. I must be making this up. I must be seeing things.

But the longer I stood there watching it happen, the smoother that area of my body became. That was when I realized the true power of gratitude and how our thoughts, feelings, and emotions create our reality. If something in your life isn't showing up the way you would like it to show up, then ask what thoughts, feelings, and emotions you have about it that is keeping it in place.

What judgments do you have about your weight, your thighs, your body, your metabolism? Judgment will always stop progress in it's tracks. Remember, your body is objective and whatever you believe about you and your body, your body will create it.

If you have been trying to change your body, get curious, ask questions, force yourself to let go of the judgments and start being grateful for your body. You don't have to fake it until you make it. Be real. Be authentic and start to find things that are actually true for you in the moment.

Can you be grateful for your smile? Your eyes? Your stomach? Your strength? Your heart? For what your bofy is truly capable of?

Pay attention and choose gratitufe.

You'd be so surprised how quickly this changes things.

Putting It into Practice

> *"When you start to have gratitude for your body, your body will do anything for you."*
> —*Katherine McIntosh*

One of my daily practices is, every morning when I wake up, I lay in bed for those first 5 minutes and go over in my head everything I did yesterday—everything my body did; every experience I had with my son, business, clients, classes. Almost always, I realize I've done way more than I give myself credit for.

It's a great way to start the day. Instead of ridicule and self-sabotage, **it's about praise, gratitude, and accomplishments.** I thank my body for everything it did for me yesterday. Then I simply ask, **What can we create today?**

That one question opens the door to something greater.

And then I pull out my journal and write down a half page to a page of everything I'm grateful for—all the things about my body, my house, my business, the earth, the people in my life. There is no right or wrong way to do gratitude. Do it for whatever is true for you and you will begin to see the world through a different lens.

You never know, your life might start to show up as if by magic. And the truth is, you *are* magic, and life is meant to be full of magic and miracles.

Bonus Putting Things Into Practice

My next suggestion may be extremely challenging for you to start. It was for me. But if you do it, it could change your entire life. It did for me.

I believe **one of the hardest things to do is to look at yourself naked in the mirror and have gratitude for every inch of your body.** Don't go into judgment. Don't go into the past. Just look at it, just look at your body, without any preconceived notion. And once you've done that, start to find all the ways you can have gratitude.

What has your body been through? Did you have a baby? What adventures have you been on? What broken bones or car crashes have you survived? Have you survived cancer? Where has your body taken you? Who have you met? What places on the planet have you seen? Who have you touched? When you begin to acknowledge that this body—*this one body* that you've been given in this lifetime—has always been here for you, you might start to treat it differently. And hey, maybe, your whole life will change.

If you are up for the challenge, I dare you, for 7 straight days, to get in front of the mirror, get naked, look at yourself, and have gratitude for every inch of your body.

And if you would like a little help taking this on, I have an amazing online course that can support and inspire you to get in front of the mirror, let go of your judgments, and express the gratitude that's possible. www.katherinemcintosh.com/ACIP

I believe that *when you start to have gratitude for your body, your body will do anything for you.* So this is your challenge...get naked, stop the judgments in their tracks, and truly find something you can be grateful for. I promise, if you do it for long enough, your life will radically shift.

Chapter 9
Play!

"The truth is that finding happiness in what you do every day is so imperative." – Gary Vaynerchuk

Here's a story to illustrate the importance of laughter and play. I was in Bahrain with a group of 30 entrepreneurs. We had just finished a week-long speaking tour with video shoots, interviews, and podcasts; we stayed up late practicing and woke up early to rehearse. It was a grueling week that left us satisfyingly exhausted. Having finished our last appointment, we got to visit with the governor of Bahrain in his Palace. We talked about the future and what we could do to make a difference in the world.

It was a huge accomplishment and honor. As the 30 of us left the palace and loaded onto our bus, I looked at my friend Patty and said, "I'm either going to laugh my ass off or cry my eyes out." The emotions had hit me hard, and being an emotional being I tend to feel things quite deeply. She replied, "Whatever you gotta do, just make sure it's fun!"

I took a seat on the bus next to one of the event coordinators, and we were having this playful banter back and forth when he asked me something and in my reply, his facial expression was absolutely priceless. I got him good and he wasn't expecting it.

That's when I lost it.

> *"In the face of happiness, everything is possible."*
> *—Dr. Dain Heer*

A full blown fit of laughter. I literally could not stop laughing—20 minutes of stomach-ache-inducing hysterical laughing with tears, drooling, and snorting. And it was infectious. Almost everyone on the bus was in tears from laughing so hard.

We had just completed 10 days of intense travel, seeing these magnificent places, palaces, the Burj Al Arab, the Burj Khalifa, meeting the governor of Bahrain, speaking on stages, connecting with change makers from everywhere on the planet…all while enduring this silent pressure to perform, grow beyond our comfort zone, and get out of our own way. The intensity of the trip came out of me, then all of us, in a giant, unexpected fit of laughter.

It was a moment of 'Uē – "oo-wēh"—the Hawaiian word that means to laugh so hard you start crying, or cry so hard you start laughing. Hawaiians believe that any healthy, sane adult should have at least one oo-weh experience a week. Children experience this state almost every day.

Yet, the *Diagnostic and Statistical Manual of Mental Disorders* the Psychiatry Bible called the *DSM* for short considers the qualities of *oo-weh* to be a psychotic state that may need medicating.

I think it's pretty insane to think that laughter and joy might need medicating. Something is very wrong here. I grew up as someone who loves to laugh, and when I laugh others around me can't help but start laughing, too. But for a good part of my life there was always this little voice in the back of my head whispering that having too much fun isn't appropriate. Life is supposed to be serious.

I don't know about you, but I think that is just a bunch of hogwash. **Life is meant to be enjoyed!** Life is meant to be fun, an experience full of surprises. And maybe give some thought to how your body came here to have fun *with* you!

So, let your hair down! Laugh so hard you start to cry, laugh so hard you start to snort, laugh so hard you start to drool because you *just can't help it*.

In those kinds of absolutely blissed-out moments, are you thinking about your thighs? Or that you had one bite too many? Or obsessively worrying about work?

NO!

Why?

When we are so immersed in the moment, there is absolutely no room for judgment.

None.

Zilch.

Which makes it very reasonable to get out and play and be immersed in the moment. Money follows joy. When you are truly being happy, you change the planet, you heal the earth, you inspire those around you, you attract even more experiences that help fuel your desire to truly have a life and living that inspires you.

Diets are not inspiring. But knowing what's true for you, developing a relationship with your body that inspires you, having those light bulb moments that no one can take away from you…

Those are the moments that dreams are made of. Those are the moments where relationships thrive, and people will start to look at you and wonder, what the heck is she doing? Just like Meg Ryan in the movie When Harry Met Sally and she loudly displays faking an orgasm in a diner and the lady next to her tells the waitress: "I'll have what she's having!" People will begin to want what you have.

It's time to stop restricting and instead start adding to your life. Add more water, more movement, more vegetables, more play, more fun, incredible friends, new experiences. Find the new, open your new neural pathways and retrain your brain for the joy of living! When you are having fun and inspired by life, you eat better, you make better life choices, but it also physically and chemically affects your body. Your metabolism can increase, your digestion can improve, your energy can increase, you can begin to appear younger, and have a healthy glow. Inspiration is not only contagious, it's healing. Your relationships will improve, your parenting will get better, your business will grow, and you will have a newfound energy for living!

Life is too short to be serious all the time and to be a constant problem solver. When you focus on your problems and are serious about those problems, you have to create more problems so you always have something to do.

Let me give you an example of how play can also be very healing. Years ago I was facilitating a retreat in Costa Rica. There was this woman who came and she was such a badass. She had a black belt and owned a Judo studio in Colorado. If I was ever in a dark alley or found myself in a situation where I didn't feel safe, I would want this woman by my side.

But Megan had a deep dark secret where she did not feel safe. She had a debilitating fear of heights. Like so deeply rooted in her reptilian brain that in college she had to get rescued by police and fire firefighters off a bunk bed in college. I also believe that whatever was stuck in her need to survive also played a role in her lifelong struggle with her weight.

Megan was strong as nails. She was fierce, kind, smart, powerful, successful, and in almost every other area of her life, she was fearless. We were processing some of the unconscious traumas that keep us stuck, while simultaneously engaging in some physical activities that would unlock the trauma in the body. Healing doesn't have to be serious. Change doesn't have to be hard. This is about letting go of all the ways you think you need to do something and opening up to the playful, surprising ways in which play can lead to profound healing and transformation.

When I started hiring "experts" to help me grow my business, I started to take my business way too seriously. Looking back, I thought that taking my business to the next level required a level of maturity that didn't involve the fun joyful ways of creating a business. The problem was, what made my business successful from the beginning was my ability to play. I took serious subjects and I made them fun and playful and people began to feel attracted to this new way of changing their bodies and their lives. It worked. It was easy. My business flourished in that environment. When I made my business serious, it began to suffer. It was no fun for anyone including me.

I had to get back to the memory of the fun. I had to reconnect with the joy of transformation, not get caught up in the seriousness of it. Many people take losing weight very seriously because they've decided it has to be hard. They think: If it hasn't yet happened after years of trying diets, pills, fitness protocols, gyms, health advice, then clearly it has to be hard. But the truth is, it is actually easy when you begin to realize that you have all the answers inside of you to unleash that brilliant, beautiful, potent, sexy, kind, energetic beast called you.

Going back to Megan's story, let's illustrate how play led this woman to literally change the course of her life and heal a trauma that was so deeply rooted in her body, she had no idea the impact it was having on every area of her life, until that fateful day in Costa Rica where she made a choice that surprised everyone.

Sitting in this intimate circle with a group of women who were eager to change, Megan told of her extreme fear of heights and shared that she wouldn't be zip lining with us the next day. She went into the story, the pain, and the fear. Her body was visibly showing signs of how and where the trauma was locked in her body. We understood her reasoning and left it at that.

We went around the circle and other women processed and healed some profound stuff. She watched women (whom she had known for years) change some things they thought they would never be able to change. Megan's eyes got wide with enthusiasm, her wheels were turning and as we were closing the circle, Megan said, "I think I want to go zip lining tomorrow."

My jaw almost hit the floor. Here was this fierce, strong, independent woman who was literally taking a leap of faith. From my background in watching miracles, I knew this was possible, but I also had concern for her safety. We would be in the middle of the jungle, 300 feet above ground. Her harness would be tied to a cable by a metal clip. There would be no medics or rescue available.

So with a fierce intensity, I looked at her and said: "Are you sure!?" She had never been more sure of anything! I knew, in that, moment, it was now my job to support her in any way and every way I could. When you mobilize your body's fear response system into a strong will for possibility, something magical happens in the nervous system and in every cell in the body that allows for a miraculous moment to occur. That moment turns into momentum that is hard to stop, but judgment can stop momentum which is why it is so important to catch yourself every time you want to entertain judgment. It's not about not having judgment come. Judgment is everywhere. It's about being resourced enough not to act on that judgment.

Once Megan decided she was all in and there was no stopping her, we did a quick 5 - 10 minute processing and she felt sure about her decision to take a leap 300 feet over the jungle floor. It was an incredible experience I will never forget. The following day, everyone was hooked in, helmet on, harnessed, and I was standing next to Megan to support her. She wanted to go last. We did a few last minute processes. I gave her some tools to help squash the fear, and to encourage her to pay attention to the excitement.

Fear and excitement have the exact same vibration. However, since we are so programmed to label things as problems rather than possibilities, most of the time where that energy begins to vibrate in the body, people immediately assume it's fear. What I've discovered is the majority of the time, it's actually excitement. Think about it: a singer going on a big stage for the very first time making a dream come true… there is so much energy coursing through their body: blood pumping, heart pounding, palms sweating, it's an indescribable rush.

Their dream is about to come true. Is that scary? NO! It's exciting!

So as Megan was about to take this giant leap on a tiny cord 300 feet above ground, I gave her some quick tools to embrace the "excitement" that was running through her body. Most of the time in one's own healing and transformation process, what's required is a shift in perspective. A small window into cracking open the possibilities instead of shutting out the possibilities by labeling it as a problem. I went first and anxiously awaited Megan's arrival on the other side.

She was timid, nervous, excited, and probably had every energy and every emotion coursing through her veins. When she got to the platform on the other side, I could see a visible shift in her. She had literally done something she never thought she would ever do in her life. That one choice was a huge victory in rewiring her brain, and retraining her body to respond differently to her body's autonomic response system.

Megan got to the platform and we had 8 more to go! With each zipline she had more confidence, more energy, more euphoria, it was so incredible to be a part of her experience. By the last zipline, she was having so much fun that she literally scared all the sweet workers because she was coming in so fast, everyone had to clear the platform so that they could catch her.

With a smile so big it was palpable, Megan's life was forever changed. As if that wasn't enough, she wanted more! She was hooked on the adrenaline, the play, the euphoria. When you change something you spent your whole life thinking you could never change, it transforms you. It opens the door to discovering what else you can change that you thought you couldn't. It's like a miracle drug, like in the movie Limitless where Bradley Cooper was hooked on possibilities, hooked on pushing the boundaries, and hooked on discovering his own human potential.

Once Megan finished the zipline, not only was her life forever changed, but the impact it had on the rest of the group was incredible. When you witness someone changing something that was a paralyzing fear, and then they get over it in a matter of minutes... it changes you. From ziplining, we hiked for a few miles that ended in a lagoon with some cliffs. You could jump into the lagoon 60 feet up. It was so exhilarating to do that! I felt like a little kid and the joy running through everyone's body was inspiring. Megan watched me jump off this cliff, like a giddy kid who couldn't stop. I got out of the water with such exhilaration, she looked me in the eyes and said: "I want to do it!"

"OMG! Are you sure?!" I replied. The answer was obvious. I was being cautious. Being tied to a zipline was one thing, but free falling yourself 60 feet above any surface when you had to get rescued off a bunk bed by authorities... Well that was something different.

As we stood at the top of the cliff, I gave Megan some questions. I always say to people, if you're going to do something that goes against your body's autonomic response system and activates your reptilian brain and causes you to go into fight, flight, freeze or fawn, ask the questions: Will I be safe? Will I survive? Will it change something? Will it be fun?

If the answer is yes, then by all means, go for it! So as we stood at the edge of the cliff, without warning, Megan catapulted herself into the lagoon! It was such an incredible moment. Megan had been wanting to move across the country for some time now, but kept coming up with excuses as to why she couldn't, why it would be too hard, it didn't make good business sense. She had a thriving studio and so many other things going for her in Colorado, her autonomic response systems rationalized with her that moving was an irrational, unnecessary choice. Until that fateful day, everything changed. Megan returned to Colorado and made the decision to move. Within 3 months, the studio was sold, house was sold, movers in tow, and she moved 1500 miles across the country.

What's even more, is Megan has probably lost almost half her original weight. She is thriving, happy, looking fabulous, and taking each day to live her best life. That can happen in a moment. Change can truly be instantaneous. The challenge is being patient enough to see the changes manifest.

So, take your body on a date and play! Get out of your comfort zone. Challenge your old patterns and behaviors and see what can happen when you mobilize your whole body towards excitement. Some of my favorite dates ever have been dates with myself with no agenda, no need, just an invitation to go play and find joy. When you are lost in the moment, there is so much available to you, and not for one second do you think about stopping that joy so you can take a long, hard look at yourself in the mirror and judge you. Is a diet playful?

No way!

But what if changing your body could be playful, fun, exciting, and exuberant? What if you could discover new things about you you never knew existed? Have you ever gone outside your comfort zone, did something you've never done before and it awakened in you a new desire for freedom?

So get outside and play! Or go inside and play! The point is to play.

What if you took your body on a playdate for even 10 minutes each day? What would that create for you and your body? Does it want to go swing at the playground? Does it want to take a walk? Does it want to rest? Does it want to take a dance class? A singing lesson? Learn a new language? Travel to a country you've never been to before? Try a restaurant you've never gone to? What is *fun* for your body? What new neural pathways can you create by going out of your comfort zone and purposely engaging in excitement?

So often we create the idea that it's work to maintain our bodies. That it takes work to take care of our bodies. In my experience, it actually takes way more work to resist the ease of joy and play. Your body's natural state is to play. Your body's natural state is to find joy. Your body's natural state is to heal itself. Joy and laughter are the two energies that heal the earth.

So if you want to create more in your life, just say "YES" to the energy.

The earth desires your joy.

One of the participants of a class I was facilitating had an experience that shows how we can ask our bodies what they need—and then receive the body's energy, whatever it is. After the class, this participant was at home and asked her body what it would take to have more muscle. A few hours later, she started to feel really sore.

Her legs hurt, and then her butt began hurting. The pain was uncomfortable, and she started to go into the wrongness of her and her body. She was really confused as to why she was sore because she hadn't done any physical activities. The soreness didn't make sense because she was just hanging out at her house.

And then she broke out laughing. Why was she sore? Because she had asked her body for *more muscle*, and building muscle usually involves some soreness.

Your body truly desires to contribute to you. It desires to give you what you ask for. What could you start asking your body for? What if you asked your body to play with the energy of aliveness? What if you asked your body to be sexy? To be lit up? To have more energy? To feel alive? To be happy doing what you love? To show you more joy? To have more money? What if your body would like to PLAY with you every day to create the life of your dreams? And what are all the ways you could play with it?

Chapter 10
Be Excited!

"The way you get to your dream life, is you continue to pay attention to that which energizes you."
—*Katherine McIntosh*

Can you imagine what it would be like if you were excited about your body?

Think about how, when you are excited, your mood changes, your body chemistry changes, you have more energy, you see the world differently, and there is a sense of anticipation that engages your entire being.

Think about some moments in your life when you had this kind of anticipatory, sweaty palms excitement. Start writing them down in the space below. Maybe it was your first date with your spouse, getting pregnant for the first time, the birth of your first child, the launch of your first business, the launch of your first book, meeting someone you admire. Maybe it was going skydiving, accomplishing something you've always wanted to do, running a marathon.

There is no right or wrong experience; this is your journey. When you write them down, try to notice how remembering those times in your life allows your body to energetically relive the moment. And when you relive the moment you change your body's chemistry. Allow those energies to move through you and inspire you. Mobilize change by re-remembering all the experiences that literally changed the chemistry and physiology in your body, just like Megan's experience in the previous chapter. Write them down and refer to this list often! It will give your body the excitement and you never know what can happen when you're excited!

_____

_____

_____

_____

_____

_____

_____

_____

Whenever I am in a place where I need to shift my energy, I recall a specific memory from my soccer days. Here's one I frequently go to in order to help shift my energy: There I was on the field, my senior year in highschool, potentially the last game of my highschool soccer career, in a stadium full of a thousand people. The score was 1-1 with 3 minutes left in the game. I knew that if we went to a shootout the other team had a higher chance of winning. I didn't want to take that risk. A deep, guttural knowing came over me, I became possessed, and I knew that whatever it took I was going to do absolutely everything in my power to win the game.

The stadium went silent. I could hear my breathing and my heart beating. As I took in this physical experience of my entire body getting so present, nothing could take me out of this piercing awareness. I saw the ball soaring in the air and ran toward it. I got it, with an opponent right on my ass (to this day I can still see her face). My heart was racing, my adrenaline pumping. The game was on the line. I started to dribble towards the goal. My opponent attacked the ball, and we both fell to the ground. I didn't hesitate, and within a half a second I was up and dribbling towards the goal while my opponent was still laying on the ground behind me. It was just me and the goalie, and I knew that, with so little time left, the ball had to go in. I took a strike with everything in me, and my foot made this perfect contact with the ball, I could just feel it. We all watched the ball soar past the goalie and into the net.

GOAL!

The crowd went wild! A roar of ecstasy came over the entire stadium. My body was completely buzzing from the euphoric excitement.

My team erupted in celebratory elation, and I was the hero.

That moment is one of my claim-to-fame moments. Our team went on to win the state championship the next day. I rely on that moment quite often to take me out of a funk, to inspire me into action, and to tap into that *anything is possible* mentality. Whenever I'm getting ready for a big event, or meeting someone important, I recall that moment from my memory banks and it immediately shifts everything in my physiology. Those are the moments that miracles are made of. It's not luck, it's purposefully recalling an emotion that literally changes the physiology of every cell in my body.

Now imagine, I was going on stage, or having a big interview, and instead of recalling that memory, I started to go down the rabbit hole of fear. What if I mess up? What if I don't say the right thing? What if I embarrass myself? Do you see how quickly we can make a choice to change any situation at any time? Megan didn't have to make the choice to go ziplining, but she had been preparing for that moment her whole life. She made the choice and her whole life changed because of it.

We are not at the effect of fear unless we choose to be at the effect of fear. We are not at the effect of our reactions, unless we allow ourselves to be at the effect of them. Part of the magic of change is being in a reactionary moment, and then taking a different course of action. We can't always prevent our reactions, they are instantaneous. But we can change the way we act after we react. It's a powerful moment when you realize you can affect your reactions and create a different outcome.

When we are excited there is an energy that runs through us that can change anything. But here's the challenge that most people face: Fear and excitement have the same vibration. The sensations that happen in the body are exactly the same. Sweaty palms, heart racing, body shakes—an intensity of energy coursing through the whole body. And most of us have been programmed to label these physical sensations as fear instead of excitement.

Think about it:

> When you go on a date, is it fear or excitement?
>
> When you leave a job, is it fear or excitement?
>
> When you go on stage for the first time, is it fear or excitement?
>
> When you teach your first class, is it fear or excitement?
>
> When you land your first big client, is it fear or excitement?

I bet if you really look at this—and answer honestly from your body, not from your head—you might be surprised that almost every experience in your life was more often excitement than fear.

We are so programmed toward fear—so programmed to go on the defense, to think about the worst-case scenario. But the reality is, the worst-case scenario rarely occurs. That means we spend a good majority of our time *worrying about a future that never happens*. When you engage in worry and fear, you take yourself out of the present moment and instead invite the past to create your future.

The body is this incredible receptor site of thoughts, feelings, and emotions. When we feed it enthusiasm, gratitude, excitement, and joy it changes the course of your future towards one that could resemble your dreams and a better life. When we feed it fear, worry, and doubt, we activate the past and recreate the past as the future. Thus creating a heavy experience.

Your thoughts create your reality. So if you decide that life is going to be hard, that no one will love you, that you'll die alone, that you'll never be able to lose weight...then you create that as your reality. And the universe will deliver experiences that are on the same vibration as your thoughts.

You get to choose.

Do you *want* to recreate the past? Or would you like to try something different by allowing yourself to choose a different way? I will tell you from personal experience that when I was suffering—when I was at the lowest points in my life, especially with my weight and my body—I was convinced there was no way I was ever going to change it.

I was correct. Because our thoughts create our reality.

Trying to talk myself into a positive spin felt nearly impossible, but it was a do-or-die moment. And so I made a demand to stop spiraling downward into the funk. I sought out the support of friends. And when I had the urge to indulge in my pity party, I stopped myself. Somewhere, deep down inside, I knew I was the only one who had the power to change me.

I also knew that, whatever it took, I *had* to change. Waking up every day hating my body, criticizing the size of my thighs, worrying about what everyone was thinking as they looked at my butt (or didn't look at my butt)...that was *not* living.

That was dying. And the truth is, I was dying inside.

If you have a point of view, your body will adapt itself to prove your point of view as correct.

I was dying inside because of endless self-criticism. I didn't even realize that I was constantly berating myself until one day in my early 30s. I was taking a class, and one evening the teacher asked me how I was. I had begun the day having a good morning, and then I started to eat and I couldn't stop. As I was eating, an outpouring of vicious thoughts came at me like a harpoon:

"You fat cow. You have no self-control. You'll never get a hold of yourself. Who do you think you are? You're not worthy of love. You'll never be able to change your body. Stop eating! Don't you have any self-control? Who do you think you are? You'll never be good enough." And on and on and on it went. It was like a self-generated tsunami that I drowned myself with. It obliterated me. And I realized that for most of my life, no matter how much I weighed, it was always there eating away at my self-esteem.

As I sat there sobbing in front of my peers, my teacher looked at me and said, **"Katherine, if you can't stop the thought, the thought isn't yours!"**

Wait—what?

It was a light bulb moment. I had never in my life been able to stop those thoughts. Like *never*. And I had always just assumed they were mine. Wait, so you mean that all those judgmental, mean, critical thoughts were never mine?

OMG.

From that moment, whenever I went down the spiral and couldn't stop it, there was some relief in knowing that the thoughts weren't mine. Now I had a way to, if not stop it entirely, at least keep it in check.

I began to know that when that voice came through me, it was as if someone else was talking to me. I started treating it like someone else speaking to me, so I would simply put my hand up and say out loud, "STOP!"

And it would stop, temporarily. Eventually, over time, that voice subsided to the point where it wasn't part of my daily experience. By continually stopping the spiral, I was able to completely change the self-generated tsunami. All it took was recognizing that we have the power to change our minds and then committing to a daily practice of confronting those self-critical thoughts. We have the power to change our thoughts. And if we're struggling to change them, well, they aren't ours. Unfortunately, most people don't recognize this. Most of us think that if we are feeling it then it is indeed ours. My experience has taught me that most anxiety, depression, pain, addiction, and eating disorders are not actually caused by the person who feels those things. Rather, those people are picking up others' thoughts, feelings, and emotions. They feel it so deeply. They think that if they can feel it, or hear it then it's theirs. That's just not true.

This is something we eventually learn over time *if* we choose it. You have to be willing to recognize that your ingrained repetitive negative thoughts are *not yours*. In order to change them, you can't just choose it once. You have to remind yourself over and over and over again. Like a new habit, you have to repeat the behavior over and over and over until it becomes a habit.

Think about anything else that takes a lot of practice or training. Someone who learns to run marathons doesn't just decide one day to run a marathon after never attempting to run before. They have to practice. They have to engage in the act of lacing up their running shoes and putting one foot in front of the other until it becomes a natural choice. In the past, when I have gotten out of shape, it's a pain to get back in.

I don't want to put in the effort or do the work because it's hard. It's uncomfortable. I'm not in shape and it takes a bit to get there. But once working out becomes a habit, I can't not do it.

Everytime you stop yourself with an excuse, stop yourself.

I had no idea that I could change these debilitating feelings that I was not enough. I thought I was doomed to a life of body torture and secretly feeling like I was not enough. But when I discovered that I could practice a different way of being every day for an entire year, I stopped the thoughts that took me down. Instead, I practiced gratitude.

The results were amazing: I had more energy. I was no longer depressed. My body dropped 2 full sizes by gaining muscle tone not by losing weight. I had a creative drive to create, and my business expanded. I started making more money doing exactly what I loved! And I was happy the vast majority of the time. I no longer spent time worrying about what to wear, and I ate whatever I wanted whenever I wanted it. The difference between me prior to starting my year-long No Judgment Diet and me after was night and day.

Not only did this change my life, I started to see how it could change others' lives.

When you let go of judgment, the body has the ability to heal itself.

I've seen people's arthritis leave after 10 debilitating years, I've seen the impact of diabetes change, I've seen depression lessen—all because people choose to no longer indulge in judgments of any kind. Judgments stop the body's natural ability to heal itself. In contrast, choosing to commit to no judgment allows the body to regenerate itself. If you don't do judgment, the body has the chance to operate at its natural, optimal state: to heal itself. Judgment compromises the health of the whole being.

Judgments are harmful, they do not generate excitement, and they are not relevant to creating your future.

Judgments are thoughts that have a very detrimental effect on the body. This can happen on a physiological level. Masaru Emoto, author of *The True Power of Water: Healing and Discovering Ourselves*, shows how thoughts affect the molecule of water. And if our bodies are composed of mostly water then every thought we think can have a pretty big impact on the health of our bodies.

I believe that constantly judging that you *should* eat salad, that you have a slow metabolism, that you're big boned…has a far worse effect on the body than if you allow yourself to fully enjoy the pure indulgence of a piece of chocolate cake that you've been craving. Eat the cake. Don't judge you or the cake and just enjoy every moment.

Avoiding is judgment. Resisting is judgment. Thinking your body will look sexy only if you only eat greens, that's judgment.

If you are one of those people who tries to eat as little as possible and still can't lose weight, I'm here to tell you that it's not about the food! Your judgments are creating your body. Your judgments are keeping your body from shaping itself in a way that would work for both of you.

Every moment of every day is a chance to choose to no longer function from judgment. When you stop functioning from judgment, your whole life can change. But the point is, you have to choose. You have to be in a continuous state of choice and action. You have to choose to no longer indulge in the thoughts and feelings that create sadness, depression, lack, and not enough.

A marathon runner who stops running and stops taking care of their body will eventually create a body that won't work as well for marathon running. It's the same way with these tools. If you stop using them you might end up back where you started. So find what works for you and do it as much as possible.

Being happy with your body is a long term commitment to choice. Every single day, you must choose that which engages your body, including movement, appreciating the taste of food, and listening to what would actually work for your body (instead of what you think will work). It's not a choose-once-and-all-will-work-out kind of thing. Imagine if a marathon runner had the mentality that he only had to run once and that should be enough.

Life is a choice every moment of every day.

Instead of looking backwards asking for what you can change, look forward and ask for what you can choose.

We have to choose. And in order to choose in a way that forms a long-lasting relationship with your body—one that is healthy, vibrant, alive, and sustains the test of time—we need to recognize the body is not a thing we choose once. It is an ever-changing, ever-choosing experience. **When you truly know your body, not from conclusions or expectations but when you begin to develop a sustainable relationship with it by asking it questions, listening to it, negotiating with**

it, and having gratitude for it, then you can create with it through the good times and the bad.

The relationship becomes sustainable when you trust that your body has your back. And it will do amazing things for you when it knows you trust it.

When I started this journey, I was constantly searching for the next solution. I would find something that promised to take my fat away and have me looking like the picture-perfect version of myself that I had decided would finally bring me peace and happiness. I would spend any amount of money on absolutely anything if I thought there was *any* chance it would work. It was absurd, yet so many of us suffer in this way. It was absurd because somewhere I knew that none of these "solutions" would work. But I was desperate, and when we're desperate we tend to look outside ourselves for answers.

Twenty years and $250,000 later I finally discovered the truth:

The answer is inside of you.

There is no answer outside of you. You know. You've always known. You are the expert. No one has been with your body in the way you have. No one knows your thoughts, feelings, emotions, fears, scars, bumps, bruises, dreams and hiccups in the same way you do. *No one* knows better about you and your body than you do. But most of us were never taught that we could be our own expert.

During my pregnancy I took a very non-traditional route, trusting that

I knew my body. When I was 38 weeks pregnant and there was a chance my due date was incorrect, I went to the hospital to get my very first ultrasound. The doctor had a horrified look on his face.

He seemed to be saying, "How could a 36 year old woman—almost 37—go this long without an ultrasound?" To him it was like I was an alien. And then he proceeded to tell me what I needed to do to prepare for the birth. I kept a straight face, but inside I was smiling…

A 50-something male doctor is going to tell me how to have a baby?

And then he was even more horrified to learn that I was planning on delivering this baby at home. I looked at him with a polite smile and just said, "I am grateful I have so many good doctors looking out for me. I live 5 minutes from this hospital, and I won't hesitate to come in if we have to."

I went on my way and ended up delivering, in the comfort of my own home, a red-headed, blue-eyed, freckled-faced wonder.

I've discovered that when I ask my body tons of questions and get really curious about what it likes everyday, it gives me the energy of what it desires. I don't have to guess; I can just begin to play with all the wants, desires, and needs that it has! When we don't come to any conclusions about the body's desires and instead truly enter into the exploration of each day, that excitement translates into more energy with the body.

Energy and excitement changes everything. Have you ever been on a date with someone and you couldn't eat? It wasn't that you were trying not to, it was that there was so much energy and excitement flying around that you didn't even think about food.

I remember one date like that. After three hours of sitting next to each other and sharing stories, we had completely forgotten about the appetizer that sat in front of us. Neither of us ate because we were so engrossed in engaging with the other. The curiosity and exploration was exhilarating! That man became my husband and the father of my son.

When we treat our bodies with that much curiosity, they begin to buzz with excitement and possibilities and will contribute to us day after day. When we show our bodies excitement and gratitude, they turn on and turn up for us to PLAY.

I've heard that the mitochondria in the cells of one body have so much energy that they could light up New York City for an entire month! That's *a lot* of energy. I wonder if you tapped into the unlimited resources in your body, how much energy you'd have to create the life of your dreams...

Chapter 11
Let go of conclusions!

"We create our own jails and live within it."
—*Gary Vaynerchuck*

Right now, how many conclusions do you have about what your body should look like, feel like, and function like? Do those conclusions create or kill your body? Do they make you happier or less happy? What would it be like to let go of those conclusions?

Do you know what your body wants?

My experience has been that when you come to a conclusion about your body, your body resists the change. If you conclude that your body needs to lose weight, what happens? Is it happy to just start losing weight, or does it hang on and resist losing weight? Usually it hangs on and resists losing weight. Most people come to a conclusion about losing weight. They decide they need to eat less, cut out, restrict, add, change, workout harder, but honestly, more times than not, those are all conclusions that rarely ever work long term.

Conclusions are dense, heavy, and weigh a lot. There is no room for growth. There is no curiosity, no possibility, no open door. Most diets are a conclusion of what will work. Eat this and this will happen. Don't eat this and this will happen. Sleep, exercise, drink water and this will happen. There is no question. A diet is one person's version of what worked for them. You have to be willing to ask: Will this work for me? What part of this will work? What part won't work.

In order for you to have true lasting happiness and success with your body and every other area of your life, you have to be willing to be curious, ask questions, and let go of all the conclusions you have. When you say this will make me lose weight, is that a question or a conclusion? When you say strawberries are good for you, is that a question or a conclusion? When you say you need to lose weight, is that a question or a conclusion?

Questions open up the door to possibilities. Conclusions close the door to possibilities. When you say you can't, you are correct. When you say you can, you are correct. However, when you ask: what would it take to create a phenomenal relationship with food and my body? Is that a different way of inviting a possibility you never before considered? The thing about a question that is truly extraordinary, is that you don't need to figure out the answer, a question opens the door for the universe to contribute to you! A conclusion usually means you have to do it all on your own.

Stop saying you can't and start asking, what can you do? What can you add to your life? What can you add to your daily regiment? Could you add in more water every day? Could you add lemons to hot water in the morning or at night before bed? What if you added cayenne and cinnamon to your hot water? Could you add in a 30 minute walk every day? Perhaps more cardio? Maybe you could find ways to add in more play?

Notice how much different that is than making the assumption that you have to cut things out in order to lose? No one likes to lose. But what could you gain? What if you could gain confidence? What if you could gain happiness? What if you could gain peace of mind?

When I first moved to Boulder, it was a very health-conscious place. As I got used to living there, I changed my diet pretty quickly and I started eating raw kale with flaxseed oil, drinking hot lemon water and straight cranberry juice. I danced and exercised at least 2-3 hours a day. I was in the conclusion that if I ate all the right things and worked my body hard then I would be healthier and my body would lose weight. What happened was the exact opposite...I gained 15 pounds. Because I didn't yet know how detrimental conclusions and judgments can be, the weight gain didn't make any sense to me. I remember being so frustrated.

From a typical diet, health, and fitness perspective, I was doing everything right. But what most diets and weight change programs don't look at is what is underneath the surface. It's those hidden subconscious thoughts, feelings, and emotions that more often than not sabotage any efforts towards success. It isn't just about what we are or are not eating, how much we are or aren't exercising. So much of it has to do with what's underneath the surface. I had become emotionally hardened—*convinced* I was doing it *right*—while simultaneously feeling inadequate, overweight, unfit, and unhealthy in my environment. I spent a lot of time comparing myself and my body to others. It's those subconscious, hidden factors that most likely played a role in why my body reacted the way it did.

I now know that I was trying to get myself healthy while concluding that I was doing it the right way. But I never asked my body if that was what it wanted in order to create lightness, joy, and possibility. I never asked what it wanted. I never asked what was *fun* for my body. I discovered that I was consuming a few things that I watched "the healthy people" consume and I never bothered to ask if it would be good for me. Turns out, those "healthy" foods were the cause of my unexplainable 15 pound weight gain.

Everytime we create conclusions, we eliminate a different possibility from showing up.

A few years after my kale-and-flaxseed-oil weight gain, I looked back on how many times in my life I had tried to eat the right things and exercise the right amount. There were so many times that I did all the "right" things, yet somehow my size was well above my comfort zone.

Finally, I realized that the only constant in what I ate or didn't eat, how much I exercised or didn't exercise, was my judgment…**I was still judging me for never being the size or shape I wanted to be.**

If you didn't buy your judgments as real, how much space would you have in your life?

Space really does create…so what could you create now?

When you are invested in creating your future, you don't have time or energy to judge you. That creative energy is forward-thinking, possibility generating, and when you are functioning from that place there is so much available to you. Why would you go back and judge you? The only reason we choose judgment is to stop the forward momentum and perpetuate the addiction to judgment.

If you've ever been in a relationship for a long time, you might know the feeling of curiosity and excitement slowly seeping out of the relationship while conclusion, judgment, and blame all start to creep in. I don't know about you, but it's never created more in the relationship if I or the other person is throwing around conclusions as if they know the answer.

I did this so many times. I even had fights where I would just tell the other person what they should say and then all would be resolved. Ain't that a joke! Obviously it never worked.

When you let go of conclusion in your relationships with people and your body, things change drastically. If you actually *ask* the body, from a sense of space and curiosity, what it wants, then just like a conversation with a loved one who surprises you with their kindness, caring, or gentleness, the body too can surprise you.

I know my body is full of surprises. Several years ago, when I had just started discovering how a life of no judgment with my body could transform my life, I was convinced I loved strawberries. In the middle of teaching a class, I was showing everyone how to see if your body desires or doesn't desire certain foods. I had some strawberries and we used them to demonstrate how you could use your body to discover what foods were good for it and what foods weren't.

I had made the conclusion that my body loves strawberries. "They're good for you," I had told myself. "They have lots of vitamins and nutrients in them." Sure enough, as I stood in front of the class asking my body if it wanted these strawberries, my body responded with a very loud NO!

Wait, body, are you sure? I thought there must have been some mistake because... strawberries are GOOD for you. So I asked my body several times more, and each time it was a clear NO! The class had a really good laugh. I was honestly in shock and it was perfect to demonstrate how you never know what foods will work for your body and which foods won't. After that experience I stopped eating strawberries all together and this "puff" I had always had most of my life subsided after 30 days. It felt as if I had lost 10 pounds. It's a perfect example of how not all healthy foods are healthy for your body. You never know what your body truly desires until you come out of conclusion and into curiosity.

Coming out of conclusion is powerful. Once, while traveling in Australia I thought (read: concluded) that my body was jet lagged. I was in Melbourne, coming from the airport, and feeling quite lethargic. Then I asked my body, "What do you know? What do you require?" Before I could sense the answer, the driver got lost and we ended up in a beautiful area of open land, with ponds and lots of space, that she didn't even know was there. We laughed, and within minutes I had a giant burst of energy and felt super energized.

When we come to the conclusion that our bodies are jet lagged or tired or thirsty or hungry *without asking*, we impose on the body our points of views about what it needs instead of inviting it to contribute its awarenesses, desires, and lightness.

After that experience in Melbourne, I thanked my body and the earth. In fact, I didn't experience much jet lag at all. The body is an amazing, resilient resource that will do everything it can to give us the energy, nourishment, and rest it needs. All we have to do is let go of the conclusions and get into the space of possibility.

When you find yourself in conclusion, here are some possible questions to ask:

Body, what do you want?

Body, how do you want to move?

Body, what would light you up and give you more energy?

Body, what do you know that I haven't acknowledged?

Body, what are you trying to tell me?

Body, what do you need?

Body, what would contribute to our future?

Body, what's a question we could ask to change this?

Chapter 12
Follow the Lightness

"If it is light for you, no one can tell you how to create."
— *Katherine McIntosh*

What's true for you will make you feel light; what's not true for you will make you feel heavy.

When I first started experimenting with the No Judgment Diet and the tools laid out in this book, it was all so foreign to me. I had spent my life following protocols—which, in retrospect, all felt heavy. If I didn't have a new protocol to follow, I went off the deep end. I would go on late-night supermarket runs in my hoodie, hiding my face, buying everything that was my go-to comfort food of the moment. I would run home and overindulge in those foods while simultaneously judging, ridiculing, and isolating myself.

It was my addiction to judgment that perpetuated this painful cycle. I was not fat. I was not ugly. I didn't have a weight problem. I had a judgment problem. I was a size 6. I danced, mountain biked, ran, did yoga, hiked, laughed, played, swam—and yet when I looked in the mirror I saw an unworthy, flabby, out of shape person. I felt ashamed.

I tried to cover up that shame with drugs, alcohol, jokes, and showing up as the life of the party. At times those covers worked well enough that I felt on top of the world, but the bottom of the cycle was quite debilitating and sometimes took me months to come out of.

When I read my journals from that time in my life where I was deep in my addiction to judgment, I can feel the tortured soul in me who had no idea how truly beautiful she was. During the years I was living in Boulder, one of the popular health trends—along with the previously mentioned kale and flaxseed oil—was to be gluten-free. Of course I adopted it to once again fit into the judgments.

While it is true for me that too many bread products can make me puffy, a really good homemade pasta, pastry, or piece of cake, when I'm not in judgment, is the most delicious thing. When I was in Rome, for example, I was still gluten-free so I wasn't eating pasta. Then one night I was out to dinner with a friend, and this mushroom pasta jumped out at me. It was the most delicious thing I had ever had. And the best part was, because I indulged in what would make my body happy, I had no bloating, no lethargy, no symptoms.

I learned when I go to restaurants to ask my body to pick the most delicious thing on the menu that it would like. I don't have a rule, and there aren't any restrictions; I ask and then I listen. It's when I don't listen that things get wonky.

When in Rome

Because it's a good example of what can happen when we listen to the body and let go of judgments, let me say a few more words about that mushroom pasta. I was so excited about the dish that my friend ordered the same thing.

At first bite, I was in heaven, making little noises and doing a happy dance in my chair. I was laughing in pure delight at how satisfying the meal was. We were sitting outside under a green canopy, surrounded by lush plants that served as a barricade to the public eye. I felt so cocooned and in ecstacy. When I looked at my friend, however, I realized that she was not having as much fun as I was.

In disbelief I asked, "Are you not enjoying your meal?" She answered, "I think because your body was so loud I couldn't hear what mine actually wanted." We both had a big giggle because it was true. I had given my body permission to be as loud as it needed to be so I could hear its requests. I followed what was light and discovered that my body was not very interested in the foods I thought I needed to eat in order to create a sexy body.

When I followed the lightness, my body chose the most delicious foods, I felt satisfied, and I didn't crave foods in between meals. I could go longer without eating, and I never felt like I was missing out on things. As a result, my body got happier and sexier. I didn't actually lose much weight on the scale, but I changed shape and lost 2 dress sizes.

More than Skin Deep

But it wasn't just my body that changed by following the lightness. This also applied to areas of business, friendships, and saying yes or no to people's requests of me. I started to realize how much of my life I spent saying yes to things that weren't actually light for me. Maybe it was my Catholic upbringing, but I always felt guilty saying no to people, which meant I was never actually saying YES to what was true for me and my reality.

When you say YES to what is true for you, you can start to create a phenomenal life. And that includes being happy with your body. When you're happy, you smile more. You laugh more. Your laughter heals the earth. You play more. You say yes to more things that light you up, and your confidence inspires others. When you lift your vibration you attract to you more possibilities and more experiences that match your joy.

Why wouldn't you want to find ways to make you happy?

What If you woke up every day, asked your body what it would like today, and just followed the lightness?

Instead of: What do you want to wear? Ask: What clothes would make you feel sexy, confident, alive, and excited today? (You can add anything in here that lights you up!)

Instead of: What do you want to eat? Ask: What foods would make you feel sexy? What foods would give you more energy? What foods light your whole body up? What foods would rev up your metabolism? What foods would open the door to more possibilities?

Instead of: What do you want to do? Ask: What adventures can we go on today? What energies would light you up today? Who can we talk to or where can we go to create a greater future?

Does your body light up reading this? Mine does! Your body is light, was born light, and loves to follow joy.

When you force yourself to go against what's light and true for you, it creates pain, suffering, weight gain, and inner turmoil. When I think about my experiment of giving myself freedom to eat ice cream every day, it felt light. It made absolutely no logical sense, it went against everything doctors and nutritionists say not to do, AND it was light! When I thought about doing it, it made me smile. It was so light and expansive. I felt like a sneaky little kid.

Eating ice cream for 30 days and losing 10 pounds was an anomaly in this reality. It didn't make any sense. Yet, by following the lightness of what was true for me at the time, it created so much gratitude and a sense of space and ease that it lit me up!

We often have a hard time believing things could be that easy. We think we need to make change hard, weight loss hard, success hard. But the truth is that success, weight loss, and change are easy when we are following what's light and true for us. And conventional wisdom doesn't always work. Instead of simply following what practical advice says, it's about getting in touch with your inner wisdom and following what's true for you, even when it makes absolutely no sense to other people.

That's where the magic is. And the way to find the lightness is to be without judgment. You need to be able to get in touch with your awareness. Remember that judgment and awareness cannot exist simultaneously, which is why most diets don't work. A diet is a judgment regimen that asks you to cut off your awareness and follow someone else's protocol.

So many of us have followed the protocol. Maybe you have some short-term success and lose weight and feel great, but the minute you go off the protocol you now have access to your awareness, which doesn't match the judgments and conclusions of the diet. So you go off the diet protocol hopeful that this time will be different. Through all this, you never quite tap into what's light for your body. You never quite grasp the concept of creating a relationship with your body, so when you go to indulge in that piece of cake off the diet, you start to feel guilty. Your judgmental alter ego kicks in, saying,

"This is a bad food. These foods make you fat. You're going to have to pay for this later. You better go to the gym and do an extra hour of cardio just to burn off the cake…"

And on and on and on the judgmental alter ego banters in judgment and heaviness. And you start to spiral down the rabbit hole of judgment. It has nothing to do with the fact that you ate a piece of cake and everything to do with the fact that you just opened the door to judgment taking over your awareness and taking over the lightness.

Every single time I have tried to force myself to diet it's always felt heavy and forced. It's a decision full of judgment and is not light in the least. Whenever I decided I needed to lose weight, I was judging my body and in resistance to it. It is impossible to change anything when you are in judgment and resistance.

HOWEVER, when I have total gratitude for my body, even if it's not the size or shape I desire it to be, it always shows up as lightness, my body tends to lose weight easily, and it all usually happens when I am eating my favorite foods. The trick is, I am not judging myself while eating so I don't overeat. There is no judgment of the food; I am so grateful and the flavors hit my mouth in the most incredible way.

I used to have this friend who would get mad at me at restaurants because I was the person who would wiggle, giggle, and make sounds that expressed how good the food was. There were even times, like in Rome, where I would do a little happy dance in my chair while eating.

One night, we were at our favorite restaurant and I was taking a bite of this delicious steak, cooked to perfection, with a side of a mushroom reduction and a glass of full-bodied red wine. I was in heaven and so grateful for the food, my body, this experience, the ambiance. I was taking it all in. For someone who has struggled so much with food and overeating and binging and starving, to enjoy food without judgment, to enjoy my body and my life while eating…this was a VERY BIG deal!

My friend looked at me and asked if I could stop it. And all of the sudden this wave of judgment hit me like a ton of bricks. It was one of the last meals we had together. If you have to judge me, especially when I am enjoying food and my body, then there is no room for you in my life.

The body loves to play. It loves to have fun. It loves to be in joy. When you nourish it, play with it, allow it to get fresh air, swim in the ocean, eat delicious foods, enjoy beautiful things…it lights up and has more energy.

Here's another story, kind of like my ice cream experiment. In my early 20s, I spent 3 years living in Quito, Ecuador, and when I first got there I had tons of judgment of my body. I had already spent years in therapy trying to talk away the weight I thought I needed to lose in order to feel more alive.

All the talk and judgment and criticism in the world never helped me feel light or lose weight. In fact, the opposite happened. The more

I focused on the problem, the more dense, heavy, and depressed I felt. And the more depressed I felt, the more I wanted to eat.

So when I moved to Ecuador, I was excited! It was new, alive, and freeing. I felt like I didn't have to bring the weight of my story with me. I remember walking everywhere and eating A LOT of fried food: fried rice, fried chicken, fried pork, french fries with mayonnaise. Lunches in Ecuador were huge, like 3 meals in one. What shocked me was I ended up losing a lot of weight there. Why? Because **I wasn't judging the food!** And I wasn't judging myself. It was a seriously liberating and eye-opening experience.

Until we stop judging ourselves, we don't know what's truly going to work for us and our bodies. But you probably know exactly what does not work for you. So don't come to conclusions about ice cream or fried food or anything else. Don't come to conclusions about healthy food and how it's supposed to be good for you. Question everything. Be curious. Discover what does work for you and know it is always changing. Follow what feels light, instead of what you think you should do.

Following the lightness is usually counter intuitive. But when you begin to trust you, are willing to make you the expert, then you can make a demand and go on an adventure to uncover your truth. This isn't about getting it right, this is about following the choices, the adventures, the energies, and the people that make you feel good.

One of my favorite questions to ask is: Will I be happy afterwards? Ask that for everything: Food, business meetings, doing your taxes, eating lunch, working out. When I first started running again, I hated it! It was painful to run, but I loved how I felt afterwards. I forced myself to run. It wasn't fun. I didn't enjoy the process, but I enjoyed how I felt afterwards. Start asking will I be happy afterwards? For everything. You may not enjoy the process of meditating, or doing your taxes, or eating clean, or going to bed early, or cutting out toxic behaviors, but you will enjoy how it makes you feel after you do those things.

What's true for you will make you feel light, what isn't true for you will make you feel heavy. Don't be fooled by things that you resist which may in the end be light for you. We are good at talking ourselves out of things that may "seem heavy" but in truth will create lightness. That's why asking will I be happy afterwards is a great way to truly discover your way into the truth of what you would like to create as your body, business, and life.

Putting It Into Practice

Light and Heavy with Food.

Remember how I thought I loved strawberries? Back when I first started teaching about this concept of muscle testing foods, I was in front of a room of 40 people and we were discussing how not all good foods are good for your particular body and not all bad foods are harmful. This is case by case, moment by moment. I was preparing to show them how to use their body to test their awareness. I grabbed a pint of strawberries, and without thinking about it, I started to muscle test my body's compatibility with this food I thought I loved. Lo and behold, my body was a clear no. I laughed and tried again. And again it was a no. I tried one more time (just in case) and it was a NO.

My face started to get flushed and all I could do was laugh.

It was the perfect moment to demonstrate all of the times we conclude that something is good for us when it actually isn't. It works the same way when we decide something *isn't* good for us, when in reality it won't affect the body in the way we've judged. These are clear examples of how judgment stops awareness.

You see, I had JUDGED that the strawberries were good for me. I didn't ask. I realized my body actually did not want me eating strawberries, and after I stopped eating them my whole body slimmed down and I lost that puff I never could quite get rid of. It showed me how much I took other people's advice and never actually questioned what would work for me and my body.

This is about discovering what will work for you. No one else can tell you what works for your body. But it does take practice to ask, listen, and respond. Absent of judgment. Absent of the need to be right or wrong. Absent of the need to prove. Absent of conclusions.

The Body Knows What it Knows.

Like I did with strawberries, we often conclude that a food that is supposed to be good for us, is good without questioning whether or not it is good. This is a judgment. Just because the FDA says it's good doesn't mean it's good for *you*. You never know the soil conditions, the farmers, the pesticides, or how your body responds to any particular food.

If you want to see how this can work for you, pull out of your fridge 5-10 foods you frequently eat that you've judged as good foods. And see if your body is a yes or no to those foods. (You can also do this in the grocery store too).

Hold the food at your belly and ask your body if this is a food that would contribute to the body you'd like to create. If it's a yes, most likely your body will lean forward, get a lightness to it, your eyes might light up. The body communicates in sensations, feelings, cool breezes, goosebumps, gut instinct, facial expressions, leaning forward, leaning back, crossing arms, head nods, shaking head, and so much more. So start paying attention to the ways in which your body is trying to give you an answer.

The key to experimenting with this is not to get it perfect, not to make yourself wrong, and not to judge you. Be curious and see HOW your body responds. When you first do this, try not to be so vested in the outcome and determine whether it's a yes or a no. Although it might be obvious to you right away, if it's not, don't make yourself wrong. You are learning a new language. The language of your body.

There could be certain days or in certain restaurants where a food might be a no, and then given a different day, restaurant, or environment, it's a yes. Everything is circumstantial, and this exercise is designed to keep you in constant question of what works and what doesn't work for you and your body. For example, when I am in Italy and France, bread and pasta are much gentler on my system than when I am in the States.

Once you've muscle tested 5-10 foods in your fridge that you've decided are "good" foods, go to your pantry or your freezer and find 5 foods that you've judged as "junk" or "bad" foods and do the same thing. Muscle test. And see what happens.

Most people assume ice cream is one of those foods that the body should avoid, but the truth is my body LOVES ice cream. During my month-long ice cream experiment, having given myself permission to have it, I enjoyed it so much that now I rarely crave ice cream anymore. But when I do eat it, I don't judge it, I indulge in it and I don't for a second think that the ice cream will create something physically unpleasant.

Instead, I indulge in the JOY of eating it until it's no longer joyful.

I can now have pints of ice cream in my freezer for months, which is a welcome change from my days of sneaking Ben & Jerry's pints and eating two in one sitting and then wrapping the empty pints in a garbage bag and trying to sneak them into the garbage or the dumpster without anyone seeing it.

The muscle test is designed to get you to start having a dialogue with your body so you can truly listen to its needs without a point of view. We all know how it feels to be judged or told no. And most of us probably rebelled against anyone that told us we couldn't do or have something.

The minute you tell me I can't have something, I want it. Well, when you tell yourself that your body can't have something, it wants it even more. What if nothing was off limits and everything was just a choice? Would that change the way you are with food and your body?

If you truly want to discover a different way and a different reality with your body, **remember that everything is just a choice.**

Chapter 13

Turn yourself on!

"So much energy is out there in the judgment of others. If some people used half the energy they used in judging others on looking at themselves and how to be better, the world would be a far better place."
—*Gary Vee*

There she was, this stunning, electrifying, red-headed Irish rock star. And let me tell you, she was a Rock Star. She had this entire bar in County Cork, Ireland completely packed. Everyone was mesmerized by her. There were moments when I just couldn't take my eyes off her. I still remember the sounds, the smells, the Guinness pouring from the taps, the shots of whiskey lined up along the rail of the bar, rosey-colored Irish faces with their hats, scarves, and sweaters, and the sound of jolly banter filling every crevice of that classic Irish pub.

She was an incredible singer. But there was so much more to it. She was pulling everybody in. It was incredible, and I was awestruck. There are a few people in the world who have this incredible capacity to mesmerize massive amounts of people all at once. Madonna, back in the day, was absolutely brilliant at it. Michael Jackson, Mick Jagger, Freddy Mercury, Beyonce—they all had (or have) this incredible, electrifying capacity to pull people in.

Part of that capacity comes from their entire body being turned on whether they are on stage or off stage. There is a sexualness to them that wakes up all the bodies around them. My point is that our bodies love to be turned on. And when I say turned on, I am referring to alive, awake, electric, inspired, motivated, creative, can't stop, won't stop. You see it when someone is in their creative genius. They forget to sleep, they forget to eat, their senses are heightened, they are tapped into something and aware of something far greater than themselves. This also happens when two people are in love. Sometimes they can't sleep, they can't eat, their senses are heightened, and they are tapped into a power that transcends reality.

The next time you are at a party just notice people's energy. When you are at the grocery store, coffee shop, or any other public place, just notice. Notice the people that you notice, the ones that have an energy to them that makes you look. When you look at them, does your body have a reaction? Notice the ones that are neutral, and the ones that are turned off. In my experience, it's much more rare these days to encounter people with their energy turned up and on.

When you are turned on, your creative juices are heightened, your sensory experiences are heightened, your body can operate at its optimum. Blood is pumping, cells are regenerating, metabolism is operating at full capacity, and so much more. You are more receptive, you are more open to ideas, to your awareness, to receiving money, inspiration, contributory people and so much more. It's a lot more expansive and generative for everyone when you live your life at it's fullest potential.

Weathering The Storm

At some point, you will piss your body off and it will speak up. You need to know how to navigate the moments that aren't smooth sailing. And vice versa, there will be moments your body will piss you off. We don't always get our way. That's not the point.

The point is, if we let go, if we allow, if we are patient, and if we are willing to know that on the other side of the storm is an electrifying moment that could catapult us into a whole new universe...then change becomes transcendental. And then the ups and downs with the body are just a natural course of progression towards a whole new reality.

What I will say about this, is that when you truly begin to form a nurturing, caring, creative, and expansive relationship between you and your body, your whole life can change, and the storms are not as vicious, nor do they last nearly as long.

Not too long ago, I had just finished facilitating a very intense, very beautiful, very transformative 3.5 day No Judgment Diet Workshop. It was exactly what was required and for the first time in a while, I felt myself really dive into a whole new area of living and being. There was an aliveness, an excitement, and a breath to my body that was like: oh baby! Let's do this! We had unearthed some really deep subconscious patterning and it was, to date, the most powerful 3.5 day workshop I facilitated after almost a decade of doing this work. Immediately following the completion of the workshop, I was woken up in the middle of the night by something that desperately needed to be purged out of my body.

Like an eruption out of nowhere it couldn't be stopped. I spent most of the night on the toilet purging out both ends. My body was a raging mess and something from that weekend awoke inside of me, had been buried, and physically needed to come out. I knew while it was happening that my body was attempting to get rid of some really old patterning. It was realigning itself with the new possibilities and in order to do that, it needed to purge the old. If you don't judge what is happening, there is always light after the darkness, calm after the storm, and breakthroughs after the breakdowns.

No One Likes to be an Afterthought

Your body loves to be a part of the journey, not just an afterthought. I would venture to say that no one likes to be an afterthought. Imagine if you could let your body be turned on by every choice you make. Turning yourself on is like turning the volume up on a song that you love and letting yourself be consumed by the energy of the sound, the words, the message. You can turn up the volume on your body.

Most of us are taught to turn the volume down....to dumb our bodies down. When your body is turned on and you turn the volume up, you invite other people to also step into their brilliance.

The body desires to gift you that kind of energy all the time. It isn't about putting yourself in a situation where you feel unsafe; turning yourself up and on also means that you are turning your awareness up so that you don't have to put yourself in unsafe situations. Awareness is your greatest protection. The body is a gift of supreme magnitude that truly desires to be your ally and contribute to you. If you let yourself be turned on by the magic of you and your body, I wonder what you will create?

Have fun with this energy and your awareness, and let you and your body be the gift that changes the world. Ask your body questions, be curious, and continue to explore the magic you can be to the world. This is your journey...enjoy the ride!

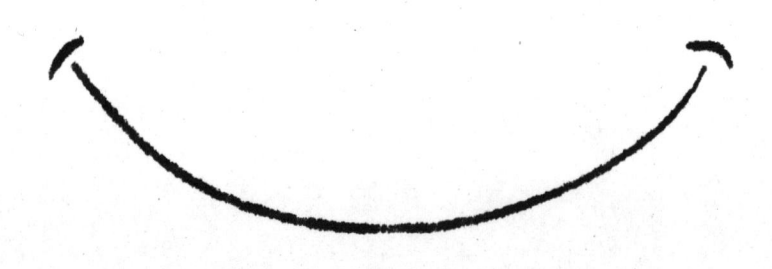

Chapter 14
Your Body's Way

You Got This!

> *"Our deepest fear is not that we are inadequate. Our deepest fear is that we are powerful beyond measure. It is our light, not our darkness that most frightens us. We ask ourselves, 'Who am I to be brilliant, gorgeous, talented, fabulous?' Actually, who are you not to be? You are a child of God. Your playing small does not serve the world. There is nothing enlightened about shrinking so that other people won't feel insecure around you. We are all meant to shine, as children do. We were born to make manifest the glory of God that is within us. It's not just in some of us; it's in everyone. And as we let our own light shine, we unconsciously give other people permission to do the*

same. As we are liberated from our own fear, our presence automatically liberates others."
—*Marianne Williamson,*

There is nothing more attractive than a person lit up by their own body and being. One who intimately knows themself and is willing to be humble, graceful, and gracious enough in their own pursuit of greatness that they leave the need to be right behind them. As one of my mentor's Gary Douglas always says: "Would you rather be right or would you rather be free?"

My hope is that you choose free. Free yourself from the self-imposed shackles of your body and give yourself permission to wake up to your body, wake up to your brilliance, and wake up to the fact that you are in charge of your own life. If something isn't working, then change it. You have the power inside of you to change that which you thought you couldn't change. It's all a matter of perspective.

No one in the world can do the work for you. No one can tell you how to be with your body. The truth is: no one in the world can make the choices you make. So this isn't just about beginning a journey in which you become the captain of your own ship. This isn't just about surviving life's challenges and storms, this is about being willing to steer yourself in the direction of your dreams.

All too often, we get watered down in our own spirit because we are too worried about what other people think. What other people think is none of your business. And sometimes, when you are in the thick of navigating your own storms, what you think is none of your business. Other people's judgments of you and your life and your choices are none of your business, just like your judgments of you are sometimes none of your business.

You are an aware, awake, bold, brilliant, beautiful being. And you deserve to be happy. Don't wait for the weight to come off to start choosing happiness. Don't wait for the money to be in the bank account to start choosing happiness. Don't assume that it's too late to get started on the life of your dreams.

It's never too late.

Be patient with yourself. Find things that you can add to your life every day that bring you joy, help you become more present with your life, and truly connect to what it is you desire to create in the world. You are unique. Your body is unique. You came into this world with your own set of physical, physiological, psychological blueprints. So you are not a one-size-fits-all body.

You are a piece of fine art, with more value than you may ever know. Start to treat yourself and your body like the unique gift it was meant to be in the world. You wouldn't buy a piece of fine art, hang it on your walls in your home, and then proceed to look at it everyday and talk shit to it. That would be absolutely absurd. So why would you do that to you?

This isn't about getting it right or being perfect in your journey, this is about discovering how to do life your way. Find ways to appreciate the uniqueness of you and your body. Develop an insatiable appetite for gratitude and appreciation. Encourage the gifts to come out, water your soul, nurture your body, and stay true to the magnificent brilliance of you. I promise you, if you stick to these processes long enough you will find the magic inside your body that works for you.

Make them yours. Use what works for you, and toss out the rest. No one can be the expert of your body. Please pay attention to the people who nurture your gifts and spirit, and whom you feel light and inspired to be around, and begin to give yourself permission to limit contact with those who bring you down.

Please know, I by no means desire to steer you from going on a diet. A meal plan, or a nutrition protocol may be the extra support you need to tip yourself over the edge to go from sluggish, lethargic, and perhaps a little defeated, to inspired, energized, and enthusiastic about life. My desire is for you to stop depending on outside advice, stop cutting off your awareness, and to become the expert of your own life. Your body is your feedback mechanism for how you're doing on your own journey. If your body is in pain, is holding onto excess weight (no matter how hard you try to lose it), then it is giving you feedback that something is off.

Pay attention. Be kind. Ask questions. Don't give up. And above all, know that you got this! When you really want something you go for it. So stop pretending that you can't go for it. You are not a victim of your body. You chose your body, your parents, your DNA, your unique blueprint. So start marveling at what this unique body and being can do. Stop focusing on what it can't do.

Wipe your slate clean, stop looking to the past for a frame of reference or proof of what did or didn't work. You are not the same person you were last week, last month, last year, so stop treating your body like it's the same. Your body and the body you truly desire to have, and the life and the business and the relationships you truly desire to have are not in the past. So stop looking there.

Start new, start fresh, begin every day like you're meeting yourself for the first time. Remember, every 24 hours 864 million old cells leave your body and 864 million new cells come into your body. Your body is not the same body that it was yesterday.

Just like your most intimate relationship, wake up and treat your body like you would the favorite person in your life. You won't get it right, but you will get it. This isn't about being right. This is about being free. Set yourself and your body free and you will be astonished at what you and your body can do.

The most valuable relationships in the world are the ones that inspire you, encourage you, lift you up, call you out on your bullshit, have allowance, gratitude, and appreciation for you, but most of all, they trust you to trust yourself. So start trusting yourself. Start trusting your body. Don't be afraid to screw it up. Stop judging you and start believing that there isn't anything you can't do. If you can't, maybe it's not because you can't, but because you don't want to. When you really really really want something, you go for it and you do whatever it takes to try to get it.

So either change what you say you want, or change your actions to match what you say you want. Pay attention to your thoughts, your words, your actions. If something isn't working, then look at what you need to change. Above all, know that no one can do your journey for you, and hopefully that excites you! Don't give up! You got this!

Appendix

Thank you for taking the time to read this book. If you are inspired and would like to further explore more possibilities that will help you wake up to the brilliant beautiful beast called your body. There is a world of possibilities awaiting you.

Here are some other ways to further explore:

Check out all the latest resources, blogs, podcast episodes, live events, classes, products and more at: www.katherinemcintosh.com

If you are interested in The No Judgment Diet online class using the tools of access consciousness, you can check out www.katherinemicntosh.com/ACIP

Let me know how this book impacted you by sending an email to katherine@katherinemcintosh.com

For information on Access Consciousness® visit: www.acccessconsciousness.com

Share on social media and write an Amazon review to help this work reach all of those who desire to change their body, business, and life.

Find me on social Media: Katherine McIntosh and The No Judgment Diet on Instagram, facebook, youtube, twitter, and even tiktok!

You can join Don't Diet Be Happy Facebook group for the latest Facebook lives and updated information.

https://www.facebook.com/groups/dontdietbehappy

Share this book with a friend

Most importantly, give yourself permission to be your own expert

You got this!

About the Author

Katherine McIntosh is a World Class Energy Worker, Global Facilitator, Author, International Speaker, and Entrepreneur. She started a multiple 6 figure business with less than $1000 to her name when her son was just 3 months old. Her business has helped change thousands of lives all over the world.

From anxiety, to stress, depression, broken bones, pain, and disease in the body to growing businesses, stepping into greatness, being vulnerable, going after one's dreams, and getting out of your comfort zone so you can live your best life, Katherine has worked with people from all walks of life from all over the world. From Hollywood Actors, Famous Musicians, World Class Healers, New York Times Best Selling Authors, to Architects, Business Owners, Speakers, Coaches, Real Estate Agents, just starting out entrepreneurs, and seekers from all walks of life looking to make their lives better.

Katherine was featured on CNBC in Dubai, spoke at both Media City and Google in Dubai, and was featured in a summit with Jack

Canfield. Katherine has facilitated classes & worked with clients all over the world including London, Paris, Rome, Dubai, Dublin, Los Angeles, Toronto, Chicago, New York City, Aspen, Sydney, Melbourne, Mexico, Bimini, and more! Katherine uses her background in somatic psychology, energy medicine, and movement therapy to invoke true lasting change in people's lives.

She treats each person from the perspective that their situation is unique. She specifically caters to the needs & desires by accessing the unknown and unwanted patterns of behavior that are underneath the surface. Through her work, she accesses these energies and helps people change them so the impact spreads to every area of someone's life.

Katherine found the power and wisdom in finding a practical and effective way to change the insecurities of her body that were holding her back from living her best life. Once she eradicated judgment from her diet she discovered the power of living by listening to her intuition. She's traveled around the world facilitating the concepts in her book that have helped thousands of people wake up to their best life. Her book Don't Diet. Be Happy is a bold, emotional, practical and personal memoir that offers tools to create your best body, business, and life by focusing on the things that really matter.

Her lifelong struggle with her body, weight, and self-image almost destroyed her. She went from a 4 time varsity soccer player with 6% body fat to someone who struggled with body dysmorphia, anorexia, bulimia and lost almost 20 years of her life. When her son was just 2 months old she had a moment in the mirror that literally changed her life.

Based on her life changing experience, Katherine learned to love the skin she was in, free herself from the mental constraints that kept her a prisoner to her own thoughts for 20 years, which allowed her to build a business she could be proud of. Once she realized the impact of these tools, she started to facilitate the exact tools that changed her life.

Katherine lives in Aspen with her son, works with clients all over the world remotely and has a private practice at The West End Med Spa in Aspen where she sees clients in person. When she's not working doing what she loves or traveling the world, she can be found skiing, snowboarding, biking, & hiking in the mountains

To follow Katherine and to check out more ways you can play with Katherine in person or online, visit www.katherinemcintosh.com

Lightning Source UK Ltd.
Milton Keynes UK
UKHW041002110722
405676UK00001B/4